NOTHING IS WITHOUT POISON

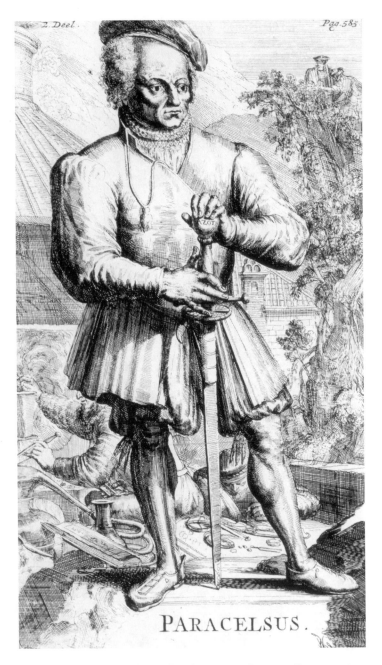

Paracelsus (1493–1541), from a Dutch seventeenth century line engraving.
(Courtesy of Wellcome Library, London.)

Nothing Is Without Poison
Understanding Drugs

Michael Roberts

The Chinese University Press

Nothing Is Without Poison: Understanding Drugs
  by Michael Roberts

ISBN 962–996–051–6

THE CHINESE UNIVERSITY PRESS
The Chinese University of Hong Kong
SHA TIN, N.T., HONG KONG
Fax: +852 2603 6692
     +852 2603 7355
E-mail: cup@cuhk.edu.hk
Web-site: www.chineseupress.com

Printed in Hong Kong

To

Dr. Henry Adam

friend and mentor for many years,
whose knowledge and wisdom sustained me
at the start of my career in pharmacological teaching and research.

Contents

Preface

Most of us experience, sooner or later, the curative or alleviative effects of modern drugs. We know, too, that many of these potent medications may cause unwanted and unpleasant toxicities, even death. There is today considerable public interest in new drug therapies and in the progress of medical science in general, but we read all too often about therapeutic disappointments and unexpected disasters.

There is also much concern about the devastating social problems of chemical abuse and addiction, where agents that lead to alterations in mood and behaviour are exploited thoughtlessly for so-called recreational purposes.

Part of the same problem is the widespread pollution in advanced technological societies of our soil, air and water by the chemicals produced intentionally or as waste products by industry.

If we are to have rational and well-informed views on all these problems, we need to know more about recent advances in the study of the way chemical substances can influence human bodily health and function, i.e., the sciences of pharmacology and toxicology. This book, therefore, aims to provide the reader with a simple explanation of some of the fundamental principles of those sciences. It sketches the history of drug treatment from traditional therapy with mainly herbal preparations to today's explosion of synthetic drugs. It outlines the roles of the academic research laboratories and the pharmaceutical industry in the development, synthesis, testing and marketing of new drugs. What happens to these drugs when introduced into the body, and how they produce their actions, the good, the bad and the fatal, are the main themes of the first part of this book.

The second part is devoted to chemical substances that act on the nervous system, as these include the drugs which are widely abused and can lead to chemical dependence and addiction. Substances acting on the involuntary part of the central nervous system (the autonomic nervous system) which controls blood pressure, cardiac function, respiration, etc., are mentioned, since their modes of action throw light on those chemicals which influence the higher centres, leading to alterations in sensation, mood, behaviour and consciousness.

This is not intended as a textbook of pharmacology or toxicology, and there is no attempt to discuss systematically all the drugs and chemicals at large in our society. However, some common ones are mentioned in order to illustrate the general mechanisms of action.

There are many reasons why the layman should be better informed about what happens, or may happen, when he breathes, swallows or has injected an unnatural chemical substance. He will then be able to evaluate better the often inflated or downright misleading claims made by the drug manufacturers for their over-the-counter preparations. When sick, he is more likely to understand what his physician is trying to do with prescription drugs, and will no longer demand the traditional role of the doctor as priest-magician. His views on the social problems raised by the use of addictive and recreational drugs, and by industrial pollutants, will be more soundly based on fact and understanding.

We must remind the reader, however, that medical treatment in general, and the sciences of pharmacology and therapeutics in particular, are today undergoing unprecedented and exciting revolutionary advances, especially in the fields of gene therapy and computer-aided drug design (see Introduction, pp. 9–10; Chap. 2, p. 22). The completion in 2000 of the human genome project opens up extraordinary prospects for new treatments based on pharmacogenomic principles. The hope is that such treatments may avoid some of the dangers and pitfalls that have bedevilled twentieth century therapeutics. Nevertheless, much twenty-first century drug treatment will surely continue on much the same lines as in the past for many decades to come. Therefore, the title of this book still remains relevant.

This book, therefore, should contribute something towards the better education of the general public and those involved in the paramedical professions in matters concerning drugs and chemicals of every provenance and application.

Michael Roberts
Albuquerque, NM, USA

December 2001

Acknowledgements

I would like to express my gratitude to Emeritus Professor Stanley Feldman, recently Professor of Anaesthetics at the Westminster and Chelsea Hospital School of Medicine, University of London, for reading the manuscript and suggesting ways of updating and improving its factual content. The final text is a much better one than it would have been without the benefit of his wide knowledge and experience. Errors and omissions that remain are, of course, entirely my responsibility.

I must also record my thanks to my friend and former colleague at the Faculty of Medicine, The University of Hong Kong, Dr. Zoltan Lett, for sustaining my enthusiasm during the revision of the final text for the Chinese University Press.

Dr. Steven K. Luk, Director, and Mr. Y.K. Fung, Manager of the Editorial Division, of the Chinese University Press and their staff prepared the manuscript for publication, and I express my appreciation here for their patience and helpfulness during this exercise.

The Index was organized with professional expertise by my wife Ursula, who also encouraged me to write this book in the first place, but, sadly, will not see its final appearance in print.

I am grateful to Ms Catherine Sanchez for her expeditious and expert typing of the manuscript, and for the preparation of the discs for electronic transmission to the Chinese University Press; and to Joseph Roberts and Rachel Dissassa for their occasional, but much needed, computer advice and assistance.

Finally, I thank the Wellcome Library, London, for permission to reproduce the line engraving of Paracelsus in the frontispiece.

Part I

If you wish justly to explain each poison, what is there that is not poison? All things are poison, and nothing is without poison; the Dosis alone makes a thing not poison. For example, every food and every drink, if taken beyond its Dose, is poison; the result proves it. I admit also that poison is poison; that it should, however, therefore be rejected is impossible. Now since nothing exists which is not poison, why do you correct? Only in order that the poison may do no harm.

T.P. von Hohenheim (Paracelsus), *The Reply to Certain Calumniations of His Enemies: The Third Defence*

Introduction

Wonderful little our fathers knew,
Half their remedies cured you dead —
Most of their teaching was quite untrue.

Rudyard Kipling, *Our Fathers of Old*, Stanza 3.

The Chemical Basis of Life

Living beings, from the simplest unicellular organisms to man himself, depend for their continued existence on the incorporation and utilization of chemical substances, and on the energy liberated by the metabolic interactions of these substances. Chemical compounds, simple or complex, are built up from the ninety-odd naturally occurring elements ranging from hydrogen, the lightest, to uranium, whose heavy nucleus is radioactively unstable. Some cosmologists today subscribe to the so-called *anthropic principle*,[1] which claims that the physical constants of the universe at the time of its origin in the Big Bang were such that heavier elements could be formed later in substantial amounts from primordial hydrogen. Had these constants been only slightly different, life would not exist anywhere in the cosmos. From that point of view, the evolution of living organisms is no accident, but is in fact implicit in the basic physics of the universe.

Implicit or not, living organisms are nonetheless very vulnerable artefacts of chemical complexity. Their existence is confined to a very few favourable environments, and their survival has been constantly threatened there by generally harsh conditions.

Whether the seeds of life developed in the primitive environment of our planet, or were carried to it from space (in meteorites, for example) is not known.[2] Some simple amino acids, the building blocks of proteins, could have been synthesized from carbon, hydrogen, nitrogen and oxygen at an early stage in the earth's history. The simple, one-celled organisms that appeared first had to survive in oxygen-free (anaerobic) surroundings. According to the biochemist Albert Szent-Györgyi,[3] these primitive anaerobes had so great a problem in obtaining metabolic energy under such conditions that they were unable to evolve into more complex multicellular organisms. Only when oxygen (O_2) came to exist in the oceans and the atmosphere, and aerobic metabolism became established, did these organisms appear.

Oxygen, however, is a highly reactive element and the dependence of life upon it has brought its own problems. Molecular oxygen itself has free radical properties, and when physiological oxidative pathways are taking place in aerobic organisms, even more *reactive oxygen intermediates* are released. Technically, free radicals are molecules or fragments of molecules containing unpaired electrons in their outermost orbitals. In the course of evolution, only those organisms which developed a complex system of defence against life-threatening free radical reactions survived. Some biologists believe there is good evidence that a number of human diseases may originate from a breakdown in these defence mechanisms.[4]

Toxicity and possible death clearly go hand-in-hand with life from its earliest history on earth. No doubt there were many other threats to survival that were successfully overcome during the process of evolution. One such threat is relevant to understanding the human response to drugs and other chemicals. When, much later on in the earth's history, complex life forms moved from the oceans to the dry land, another major crisis arose. The evolution of land animals necessitated the development of mechanisms for the conservation of salt and water, obviously a problem of minor importance for creatures of the ocean. These mechanisms, primarily renal, had the serious disadvantage of also reabsorbing into the body toxic substances that were ingested in food and water. Continued reabsorption, or inability to excrete these substances, could lead to their accumulation to lethal levels.

Land animals, therefore, had to evolve special, but rather non-specific, enzymes to change (or metabolize) these possible toxins to harmless, or more readily excretable, derivatives . When man began to swallow natural and unnatural chemical substances for medicinal purposes, these enzymes also acted on them, with results that will be outlined later (Chap. 1, p. 14).

The higher animals also developed many other defences against external threats, e.g., clotting systems to prevent the loss of vital blood after injury; the immune system to protect against foreign proteins from viruses, bacteria, pollens, etc. All these challenges to survival, however, were dealt with by leisurely evolutionary changes in structure, function and bodily metabolism. Evolution could not, of course, start afresh at every challenge, but nevertheless showed remarkable ingenuity in modifying and adapting mechanisms that were already in existence.

Today, the most serious threats to life on earth come from man himself, who is the maker of an incredible variety of chemical substances unknown to nature. These may not only adversely affect human and animal health, but also the whole ecology of the planet, e.g., the well-known depletion of the ozone layer by chlorofluorohydrocarbons (CFS). The evolutionary process is much too slow to develop biological counter-measures in time to prevent disaster. It depends on man himself to institute global control of lethal substances and activities through social and political measures, and most observers now believe the crisis has to be taken seriously in the years to come.

Arguably, it is the medical profession that is, without malicious intent of course, the biggest purveyor of toxic chemicals to the human organism. This is known as drug treatment, and modern medicine would be the poorer without it in the cure and alleviation of disease and discomfort. But, as we shall see later, it is not unfair to regard most drug therapy as merely a form of controlled poisoning, which is, on balance, beneficial to the patient. Nevertheless, the toxicity is implicitly there however effective the treatment, and cannot be disregarded.

Traditional Medicine

Since prehistoric times, man has swallowed naturally occurring materials for purposes other than the simple satisfaction of hunger. As he roamed the forests and savannahs of the five continents, he discovered quite accidentally that certain plants and fungi were toxic and must be avoided as food. However, he soon realized that they could be used in the preparation of extracts for arrow poisons in the killing of game, and for defence against enemies. We must salute the primitive genius who later found that these natural poisons, when taken in sub-lethal amounts, had effects that could contribute something valuable to the welfare of society. These effects were: first, a curative or alleviative action on human disease, and second, the creation of unusual states of consciousness that could be exploited in religious and tribal ceremonies.

In this connection, it is significant that the Greek word *pharmakon*, which is the root of our words pharmacy, pharmaceutical and pharmacology, means not only a curative drug but also a poison, a charm, a spell or an incantation.

One can speculate endlessly on which came first, the therapeutic or the ceremonial use of poisonous plants, fungi and, less commonly, parts of animals or materials of mineral origin. But from what we know of primitive societies today, it is likely that skill in both areas came to be possessed by the medicine man, the witch doctor, the shaman or the *curandero* who, for that reason, acquired great prestige and authority in his society. In fact, the magician, the priest and the medicine man were probably often one and the same person.

According to Brian Inglis,[5] the medicine man did not usually practice medicine in the ordinary sense. He practiced magic, with healing his objective — though, as the assumption was that disease was caused by magic or witchcraft, the remedy was designed to harm the man or evil spirits causing the disease.

Nevertheless, primitive medicine knew of many plant drugs, e.g., opium, cascara, digitalis, rauwolfia, that are still used in modern therapeutics. And even today, in the rain forests of the Amazon basin and elsewhere, there are shamans with access to plants that could be valuable in medical treatment. Unfortunately, the days of these men are numbered and their knowledge, handed down no doubt through countless generations, is doomed to be lost. Attempts are being made by groups of anthropologists and doctors to preserve at least some of this knowledge. Whether their efforts are entirely worthwhile is debatable, for reasons we will discuss later (see pp. 23–24).

Moving from prehistory to recorded history, in those times when man settled more permanently in the great river valleys and developed complex civilizations, primitive medicine underwent an evolution to so-called *traditional medicine*. The more effective procedures of earlier medicine were retained; clinical and therapeutic observations were made, often with great accuracy and prescience, and recorded in written treatises. Pharmcopoeias were produced which are still extant to this day, e.g., the Egyptian Papyrus of Ebers, and the materia medica of the legendary Chinese emperor Shen Nung (actually compiled about 400 BC.)

In those times, most new therapeutic measures were stumbled upon by chance.(It is humbling to remember that even after nearly 130 years of scientific pharmacology most new drugs are discovered by trial-and-error.) But the human mind abhors the vagueness of empiricism; it prefers an explanation, however fanciful or far-fetched. The findings of traditional medicine were rationalized into highly complex and speculative systems. These rigid systems, designed to explain the nature of disease and the efficacy of therapeutic régimes, became a block to further progress. The written word gathered too great an authority, e.g., the dogmas of Galen that hamstrung European medicine until the time of Paracelsus.

This stagnation was eventually broken up by the development in Europe of organized science in general and of medical science in particular. Just as the science of chemistry in its early days drew on empirical knowledge accumulated by the alchemists, scientific treatment of disease drew on those aspects of traditional medicine practiced in Europe at that time. Certain plants or herbs with an age-long reputation have been taken over by the modern physician, but European traditional medicine has in general been pushed to the *fringe* and is readily ignored or regarded with amused superiority.

However, in certain parts of the world, e.g., India and China, some traditional medical systems still actively flourish, and retain respect and popularity even in the face of scientific medicine imported in quite recent times from the West. It is reasonable to suppose that these old-established systems may contain something of value, and should be thoroughly investigated by the methods of modern science. Since those plants yielding useful drugs tend to have a relatively narrow geographical distribution, and species and varieties differ from one continent to another, herbal pharmacopoeias obviously vary from one culture to another. This is important, as it implies the possibility of finding, even today, new pharmacologically active substances in plants used in the less well-known traditional systems

Research into traditional herbal remedies has been, and is being, carried out, and some discoveries of significance have been reported. But on the whole results have been rather disappointing. Many herbs have minimal potency even when genuinely active. Plants containing substances of higher potency have often been disseminated widely and are already well-known universally. Many plants, even of different species, appear to have similar biochemical pathways and so are liable to elaborate the same end-products. Atropine-like compounds, such as those occurring in *Atropa belladonna* or deadly nightshade, and cardiac glycosides such as digoxin, turn up in many plants all over the world, to take two simple examples.

Modern Medicine

It is, of course, the development of the pharmaceutical industry, founded on a healthy chemical industry and a knowledge of organic chemistry, that has led to the explosive growth of modern synthetic drugs. Some of these synthetic drugs are copies or modifications of known natural products, others are unique to the laboratory. Few people today are unaware of the enormous importance of modern drug therapy in the cure and alleviation of disease. But they are also concerned with the toxic effects of these chemicals, and the fact that some of them are taken for non-therapeutic purposes and can cause serious problems of abuse.

It should be understood that the three aspects of drug action — the curative, the toxic and the so-called *recreational*, which have been known since prehistoric times — all have a common source: an interference with the normal biochemical machinery of the body. Even brain function, which at one time was regarded as depending solely on the electrical activity of nerve cells (i.e., a sort of incredibly complex telephone exchange or computer), is now known to involve a plethora of chemical substances as well. As has been known for millennia, foreign chemicals can have very profound effects on the brain. These effects are due to the interference with what is called *chemical transmission* in that organ (cf. Part II).

This is true, whether the chemical comes from a plant or fungus, or from the laboratories of the pharmaceutical industry. There is no special magic about the natural substance when it comes to therapeutic efficacy or potential toxicity. The drug purified from natural sources is no different in action from the same compound synthesized by the white-coated chemist.

Yet we must admit that the plant can be a remarkably versatile manufacturer of substances that influence human physiology and biochemistry. Even primitive man must have wondered why some plants should make compounds that can cure or kill. That so many of these plants are to be found in tropical rain forests where growth is abundant and competitive would suggest that the chemicals they make are intended to poison, or at least discourage, insects, browsing animals and other predators. Not everyone agrees with this theory, and it is also possible that some of these natural substances are merely waste products of plant metabolism that happen, incidentally, to have actions on animals.

Another site of vicious chemical warfare between species is the coral reef, a marine ecosystem which occurs in shallow tropical waters between 30°N and 30°S of the Equator. Here, also, therapeutically active substances have been looked for and found.

To kill or poison, a substance must interfere seriously with physiological mechanisms. To give less than the lethal dose of that substance *may* produce alterations in function that, on balance, benefit a patient who suffers from a disease-induced abnormality. From this point of view, therapeutics must be regarded as a form of controlled poisoning in which the therapeutic agents have implicit toxicity that should not be overlooked.

It is this fact, apparently so well understood by Paracelsus many centuries ago, that underlies our discussions about drugs and chemicals in the chapters that follow.

The Future

But before we embark on our account of the therapeutic activities of present-day drugs and the toxicities which are almost inevitably associated with their administration, let us briefly outline some efforts that are already being made to eliminate, or at least greatly diminish, such adverse effects.

The problem with most drugs past and present is that they are nearly always introduced into the whole body. So they act not only where we want them to act, but elsewhere where they may produce unwanted actions. The pharmaceutical industry has attempted, with limited success, to target drugs to specific cells in the body; or to devise a proactive agent which is activated only at the required site of action, e.g., in the treatment of some types of cancer.

Fundamental improvements in therapeutic safety, however, are more likely to arise from the recent rapid developments in the science of genetics. The specific gene or genes involved in certain diseases were already being revealed even before the completion of the human genome project in 2000.[6] This raised the possibility of replacing a faulty or missing gene with a normal one. However, there are complex technical difficulties in effecting such a replacement. Also relatively few diseases depend on a single gene defect. This is the case, for example, with the rare neurological disorder known as Huntington's Chorea or Huntington's Disease, caused by a single error on chromosome 4.

Most diseases are caused by several defective genes which interact with each other and with the environment. Therefore attempts to replace faulty genes with healthy ones have not been conspicuously successful. The main applications so far of this new genetic information have been in the development of diagnostic tests for certain potential diseases, e.g., breast cancer, bowel cancer, Alzheimer's Disease. Whether patients will wish to know or be told if they carry potentially lethal genes is, of course, a matter for ethical debate.

The attempt to develop tailor-made drugs with minimal or no toxicity is being approached in several different ways. A patient's genetic make-up may determine whether a particular medication will be more or less effective, and also more or less toxic. One day a pharmacist may, after checking the patient's genetic profile, prescribe him a particular version of an antihypertensive drug, but quite a different version for another patient with high blood pressure. This will put an end to the 'one size fits all' style of prescribing that we follow today.[7] Determining whether a patient has an ineffective mutant variation of the important drug-metabolizing enzyme cytochrome P450 in the liver (see Chap. 7, p. 53) would raise a red flag not to treat that patient with drugs poorly metabolized by that enzyme. The resulting increased levels of such drugs could lead to enhanced toxicity.

The three-dimensional computer visualization of receptor sites on the proteins produced by specific genes could aid in the synthesis of specific chemical compounds that would combine with these receptors in order to promote or inhibit their normal functions (for a further description of receptor-substrate interactions, see Chap. 13). This is the new field of rational drug design or pharmacogenomics, or, since it is the proteome (the range of proteins produced by the genome) rather than the genome itself that is important in drug action, pharmacoproteomics might be a better term. As J. Craig Venter (President of Celera Genomics, the company that first completed a rough draft of the human genome) said: "Knowing the genome will change the way drug trials are done and kick off a whole new era of individualized medicine."

Progress in all these directions may in decades to come lead to a revolutionary new therapeutics without toxicity or other side effects, though experience should caution us that this goal may not be achieved without unexpected problems, even disasters. Ultimately, we can hope that one day the hit-or-miss dosage of patients with potentially toxic laboratory-synthesized chemicals will come to be regarded as the legacy of a barbaric age.

1

Cure Or Kill?

Cur'd yesterday of my disease,
I died last night of my physician.

Matthew Prior (1664–1721)

This quotation from the aptly titled poem, *The Remedy Worse Than the Disease,* indicates that the Elizabethan poet and diplomat, Matthew Prior, was well aware of the dangers of heroic medical treatments. The essentially poisonous or toxic nature of many medications, even in the old days of predominantly herbal preparations, was, of course, fully realized by Paracelsus in the sixteenth century. Unfortunately, Paracelsus' alchemical background led him to advocate alternative therapy with many inorganic substances containing mercury, lead or antimony (calomel, tartar emetic, etc.).

By the late eighteenth and early nineteenth centuries, it had become a therapeutic fashion to administer massive doses of these and other toxic chemicals, combined with blood-letting, cupping, blistering, sweating and purging. Such treatment was known as allopathy, and it led to many deaths, although the physicians claimed that *the patient died cured.* A good example of this *furor therapeuticus* was the final illness of America's first President, George Washington.[1] During the evening of Friday, 13 December 1799, after spending the previous day on horseback in rain and snow, he developed a sore throat and experienced some difficulty in breathing. A *bleeder* was sent for immediately to remove fourteen ounces of blood from Washington's arm. A posse of distinguished physicians arrived the next morning at the gentlemanly hour of 11 a.m., and ordered further copious bleeding, two doses of calomel (mercurous chloride) and a cathartic enema. Later, as (not surprisingly) his condition deteriorated, he was given a large dose of calomel together with tartar emetic (potassium antimony tartrate), and a local treatment known as *blistering* to his throat and feet. After hours of this medical torture, Washington managed to convey to his attendants that he required no further treatment, but preferred to be left to die in peace. Twenty-four hours after his initial mild symptoms, at 10 p.m., 14 December, he breathed his last.

Ironically, around the time of Washington's death, there were already the beginnings of a challenge to heroic therapy from homeopathy[2] and some other unorthodox medical systems. The Saxony-born physician, Samuel Christian Hahnemann (1755–1843), first conceived his homeopathic theories in 1786, and expounded them in detail in his book, *Organon of Homeopathic Medicine,* in 1810. The principles of his system of medicine were, first, that a disease could be cured by drugs which produced in a healthy person the symptoms associated with that disease; second, the smaller the dose of a drug, the more effective it was in curing that disease. The first principle did not have, nor could it ever have, any kind of scientific basis. It is, no doubt, the second principle that led to any success that homeopathy enjoyed in its early years. The law of infinitesimals, i.e., using extreme dilutions of drugs, at least ensured relative safety and minimal toxicity; and the well-known placebo effect (see Chap. 3, p. 29) could operate with favourable results.

Interestingly, homeopathy arrived in England with Queen Victoria's consort, Prince Albert. He brought with him an essay of Hahnemann's entitled *On Poisoning by Arsenic*, and convinced Queen Victoria of its scientific merits. Later, she persuaded the famous prime minister Benjamin Disraeli,[3] who was being treated with large doses of arsenic for his troublesome gout, to change to a homeopathic practitioner, Dr. Kidd. Disraeli died in 1881, probably from arsenic-induced kidney failure.

Even in spite of such royal patronage, homeopathy during Hahnemann's lifetime remained on the fringes of therapeutics, and it remains there today. Later in his career, from 1829 onwards, Hahnemann drifted into absurdity with his law of infinitesimals, recommending the administration of all drugs up to the thirtieth potency. This meant a dilution corresponding to one part of drug to 10^{10} parts of water. This works out at a dose content of one molecule of drug in a sphere of water with a circumference equal to that of the orbit of Neptune round the sun. Obviously, the chance of a therapeutic dose containing any drug at all would be astronomically small. In 1988 a group of French homeopaths led

by J. Benveniste claimed in the scientific journal *Nature*[4] to have shown
that a biological agent (an antiserum) had activity even when diluted
beyond the point at which any molecules of the agent would remain. The
hypothesis put forward was that the antiserum molecules left an image of
themselves on the solvent molecules (water) during the dilution
procedures. That such unlikely findings were published in *Nature* caused
much adverse criticism, and a team (including a professional magician to
smell out any possible fraud!) was sent to check the experimental
protocols. No fraud was uncovered, but the experiments were not
considered to be adequately controlled. Later Benveniste was challenged
by a popular French magazine *Science et Vie* to reproduce his results under
conditions set by the magazine. Benveniste refused, saying that his
researches were not accountable to people "not even qualified for the job
of porter" in his laboratory!

But interest in homeopathy still persists. A very recent publication in
the *British Medical Journal*[5] reports a clinical trial purporting to show that
in some allergic conditions, (allergic rhinitis) homeopathic treatment was
more effective than a placebo. However, the trial was criticized as being
too small to be regarded as conclusive.

Allopathy or heroic therapy became increasingly unpopular and by
1860 was being gradually abandoned by orthodox medicine, but drugs of
recognized toxicity continued to be used. A more balanced common-sense
view of therapeutics came to be accepted along the lines of William
Witherings's 1789 dictum: *Poisons in small doses are the best medicines;
and useful medicines in too large doses are poisonous.*

This comment, and the teaching of Paracelsus that *all things are
poison, and nothing is without poison; the Dosis alone makes a thing not
poison* is understandable when we consider that the human organism is a
highly interdependent commonwealth of individual cells whose functions
are mediated through precisely regulated levels of physiologically active
chemical substances. Even the administration in excessive amounts of a
substance as necessary for life as water can alter the internal environment
(what the most famous of French physiologists, Claude Bernard, called the
milieu intérieur) in ways that can be definitely harmful.

We may avoid the taking of drugs, but no one can live without food.
How does the body escape the potential toxicity of the many chemical
substances in our diet, however organically grown?

Of course, those components of food that are essential nutrients —
proteins, carbohydrates and fats — are broken down and incorporated into

bodily tissues. They can hardly be regarded as poisons, though an unbalanced diet (e.g., too much saturated fat), may adversely affect one's health in the long run. But nearly all foodstuffs contain many other natural chemical substances not required or utilizable by the organism, and these must be eliminated by excretion, or by chemical alteration (metabolism) mainly in the liver. The processes of excretion, and of liver metabolism brought about by specialized enzymes, are very important in the body economy. Without them, many chemicals would accumulate in our bodies and might eventually reach levels which could cause toxicity.

This problem has been intensified in our times by the addition to foodstuffs of unnatural substances such as preservatives, flavourings and dyestuffs, not to mention possible contamination with pesticides, herbicides and other chemicals used in modern agriculture and industry.

The metabolizing enzymes of the liver are versatile and can act on many different types of chemical compound, including many of the modern drugs given by the physician. The usual effect of this metabolic activity is to convert the foreign or unwanted substance into one that is less poisonous or more readily excreted from the body. Without these enzymes, treatment with certain drugs would be virtually impossible, as these agents would remain in the body for a considerable length of time (even for life, sometimes), and would, therefore, disrupt physiological function indefinitely.

Obviously, these enzymes did not evolve in anticipation of the growth of the pharmaceutical industry in the twentieth century, but had appeared much earlier in evolution to deal with natural substances in the body. Exactly when they appeared is not known, but it is possible that some at least were present before life moved from the sea to the dry land (see "Introduction"). Complex organisms need to regulate their growth and metabolism by means of endocrine glands which secrete hormones into the circulation. These hormones, often fat-soluble steroidal compounds, can be regarded as internally produced drugs, and they must be chemically-altered by enzymes if their actions are not to be unduly prolonged in the body. Many drugs given today are acted upon by these and similar enzymes.

As already mentioned (p. 4), the emergence of life forms from the ocean intensified the problem, because of the increased need to conserve salt and water. The tubules of the kidney were modified to reabsorb salt and water, and some other essential substances like glucose and amino acids. Unfortunately, other lipid (fat)-soluble substances are also liable to be reabsorbed into the circulation by these mechanisms. However, the liver enzymes can convert these lipid-soluble substances to metabolites of increased water solubility. These metabolites are no longer so readily reabsorbed through the renal tubules, but are excreted in the urine, so preventing accumulation in the body.

The metabolites are also liable to be less poisonous (though not invariably so), and for this reason the process is sometimes called *detoxification*.

Even with these built-in safeguards against prolonged retention in the body, the administration of any foreign chemical must still be regarded as a form of *internal pollution*. If it is given by a physician as a drug and if adverse or toxic effects are produced, then we can talk of an *iatrogenic disease* (Iatrogenic means caused by a doctor). Iatrogenic disease is widespread today, especially among hospital in-patients who are liable to be prescribed a multiplicity of drugs. The record is said to be 41 different drugs received by a patient during a single admission to a hospital in London, England. It was estimated many years ago at Johns Hopkins Hospital in Baltimore, MD, that the recovery of one patient in every five was delayed by drug toxicity. Among the seriously sick elderly, there is a definite mortality from drugs given in hospitals; an exact figure is difficult to establish, for obvious reasons, but 0.3% (three deaths per 1000 patients) has been suggested.[6]

This situation is one of the results of the *drug explosion* of the past fifty to sixty years. The carefully selected, *tailor-made* drugs produced by the pharmaceutical industry are, as a rule, more potent than the older *materia medica*. They interact more specifically and more effectively with cellular function; but, for that very reason, they are more liable to cause toxicity and other undesirable actions. Let us see why.

In a disease which is caused by some disorder or aberration in the functioning of certain cells in the body, it is difficult to conceive in most cases how a foreign chemical substance could restore cellular function to a state of true normality. In fact, more often the drug produces in those, or other groups of, cells some compensatory cellular abnormality which, in combination with the existing defect, happens more or less to mimic normality. This, however, is not restoration to a state of true health.

For example, in heart failure, a disorder in cardiac function may lead, by a series of processes, to retention of salt (mainly sodium chloride) and water in the tissues (oedema). One common therapeutic measure is to give a drug which stimulates urine flow (a diuretic), and thereby promote the loss of salt and water from the tissues. The diuretic does not restore normal cardiac function, and the *cure* is really the induction of an approximately compensatory abnormality in the handling of salt and water by the cells of the kidneys.

From this point of view (as mentioned in the "Introduction"), much drug therapy is clearly a form of selective toxicity which the physician regards as advantageous on balance to the patient in relieving his symptoms (or some of them, at least). Meanwhile the doctor waits for the *vis medicatrix naturae* (healing power of nature) to restore true health, at which point the drug or selective poison can be stopped.

These pessimistic, even somewhat cynical, remarks do not necessarily apply to all types of drugs used in medicine. Those which are given, not to influence body cells, but to eliminate invading organisms such as bacteria, are known as chemotherapeutic agents or antibiotics. Here the aim is selective toxicity against the foreign cells combined with harmlessness to the body's cells (cf. Ehrilich's search for the *magic bullet* against syphilis). This has been virtually achieved with benzylpenicillin which is one of the least toxic antibiotics known, though, rarely, it can cause sensitivity reactions. There is no guarantee, however, that a drug which can selectively kill bacteria by one action may not have other actions on human cells based on quite different mechanisms. These other actions could lead to marked toxicity, and most antibiotics discovered since penicillin have been found to be far from harmless to the patient. Nevertheless, the discovery of increasingly selective agents for the treatment of infective diseases has been one of the most striking medical advances of the last century, and has played a vital role in dramatically improving health and longevity.

Drugs given not to treat disease, but to alter bodily function and sensation, e.g., muscle relaxants, sleeping pills (hypnotics), pain-killers (analgesics), local and general anaesthetics, exert their actions on normal cells. These actions are a kind of poisoning also, but such drugs are generally given for a limited time only and, when they are withdrawn, the subject's cells should quickly return to normal. But, again, the drug may have more than one kind of action, and the other actions can be harmful, e. g., certain general anaesthetics may have long-term toxic effects on the liver cells.

The replacement of certain vitamins and hormones in states of deficiency (e.g., vitamin C for scurvy or insulin for diabetes mellitus), is obviously a kind of therapy which approximates quite closely to the ideal of restoring cellular normality and good health. In replacement therapy, therefore, one would expect toxicity or side effects to be absent or slight, since the agents given are normally present in the body and are necessary for health. The chemist Linus Pauling, who twice won a Nobel prize, coined the term "orthomolecular medicine" for this system of preserving health and curing disease by increasing the amount in the body of substances normally there. He dismissed conventional treatments using foreign chemicals, with considerable justification, as toximolecular medicine.[7]

Pauling stretched his quite logical ideas to a degree which antagonized the medical establishment, e.g., megavitamin therapy using massive doses of vitamin C (10G/day upwards) for cancer. Since vitamins are chemical substances that need to be ingested in our food (because the human organism cannot synthesize them in adequate amounts), Pauling's megadose administration of these natural substances tends, like Hahnemann's infinitesimal doses, to have minimal toxicity. But one can have too much of a good thing; it is possible to take an overdose of vitamins A, D and some of the B group, with unpleasant results. Megadosage with pyridoxine (B6) may cause damage to the peripheral nerves (neurotoxicity). Goodman and Gilman report that such effects only occur with doses of 200 mg/day or more[8] (the RDA or recommended daily allowance is 2 mg/day for adult males), but occurrence of neurotoxicity at doses of over 10 mg/day has been reported.[9] However, this damage resolves when the vitamin is stopped, and, as Pauling claimed, no one ever died of poisoning by overdosage with vitamins.

The problem of repairing deficiencies of hormone secretion is a trickier one. Although it is quite possible to administer precisely the same hormone as that made in the body (e.g., human insulin manufactured by genetically-engineered bacteria; thyroxine), it is not easy to simulate the way the naturally-produced hormones are made available. Most hormones are secreted directly into the blood stream from specialized endocrine glands, and the amount secreted is exactly controlled according to physiological need by subtle feedback mechanisms. Insulin secretion from certain cells of the pancreas, for example, depends on the levels of blood glucose. Taking hormones by mouth or by injection does not imitate physiological control, and adverse results may occur with incorrect dosage, e.g., hypoglycaemic coma from too large a dose of insulin. Attempts are being made to overcome such problems by implanting ingenious devices which can monitor blood sugar levels, and then inject just the right dose of insulin required.

The fact remains, however, that the majority of drugs coming on the market today from pharmaceutical firms are the foreign chemicals so despised by Linus Pauling. These are not the traditional herbal remedies that did not kill but rarely cured, nor the inorganic chemicals of the heroic age of treatment which cured by killing, but are sophisticated organic compounds that interact with the physiological machinery of our cells to produce the specific effects required by the physician. It is to the development of the sciences of chemistry, physiology, biochemistry and pharmacology over the past 150 years that we owe the modern drug explosion, providing the essential hope of a selective and minimally toxic *pill for every ill.*

2

Science to the Rescue

[I]f the whole materia medica, as now used,
could be sunk to the bottom of the sea,
it would be all the better for mankind,
— and all the worse for the fishes!

Oliver Wendell Holmes (1891)

The American essayist and physician Oliver Wendell Holmes was referring, of course, to the materia medica contained in the official pharmacopoeias of his time. These consisted mainly of herbs and herbal extracts of ancient lineage, together with some inorganic chemicals introduced by the alchemists and the early chemists. Although some of the herbal remedies were genuinely therapeutic and are still in use today, many had little or no pharmacological activity. They depended for their efficacy, if any, on a placebo effect (Chap. 3, p. 29) reinforced by the physicianly authority with which they were prescribed and administered.

This has all changed dramatically over the past fifty to sixty years as a result of the extraordinary development of scientific pharmacology, and the technical applications of its findings by the flourishing pharmaceutical industry. Pharmacology as an academic discipline was established in Germany in the mid-nineteenth century, the first professorship being held by Oswald Schmiedeberg at the University of Strassburg (Fr. Strasbourg) in 1872.

However, even earlier, some great French physiologists had turned their attention to pharmacological problems. For example, François

Magendie in 1821 investigated the actions of a plant *Strychnos nux-vomica*, used in Java and Borneo as an arrow poison. This contains the very potent substance strychnine which has no real therapeutic value, though it used to be added in minute doses to the *tonics* freely dispensed by doctors before World War II. Claude Bernard experimented with another arrow poison, this time from South America, called curare. This substance paralyses muscles, and it, or substances with similar actions, are used today to produce relaxation during surgical anaesthesia.

There are two interesting points to note here. First, these scientists were still concerned with the natural plant drugs of traditional medicine (or perhaps one should say "traditional toxicology"). The era of chemically-synthesized drugs was some way in the future. Second, they investigated drugs not so much for their therapeutic applications, but for the light they could throw on normal physiological functions. Bernard, in particular, saw toxic substances "as kinds of physiological instruments more sensitive than our mechanical means, and well suited to act, so to say, in dissecting one by one the properties of the anatomical elements of the living organism." In other words, drugs were regarded as tools for studying normal function on the basis that, if you disrupt, slow down or stop a process, it often becomes easier to see how it was working before you interfered with it.

An increased understanding of what a drug did to the normal physiology of the body was sought in greater depth by the academic pharmacologists from 1872 onwards. Gradually a considerable body of knowledge was built up about the way drugs act. In order to place this knowledge on a sound footing, it was necessary to apply techniques from other sciences such as chemistry, biochemistry, pathology and statistics.

Chemistry made an especially important contribution. The organic chemist was recruited to make extracts of plant and animal tissues used in traditional medicine, and, if possible, to purify and identify the so-called *active principle*, i.e., the actual chemical compound or compounds responsible for the therapeutic or pharmacological action.

For example, opium, known since antiquity as a product of the white poppy *Papaver somniferum*, was extracted by the chemists, and one of its active principles, morphine, was isolated in pure crystalline form. This, in itself, was a great advance. Instead of a plant product (opium resin) of unknown composition and variable strength, we have a pure active substance which can be weighed out for precise dosage. Pure solutions of morphine salts can be sterilized and put into ampoules for injection. (This is not an unmixed blessing, though. The immediate onset of action after injection facilitates the establishment of a state of addiction.)

Many other active principles from plants (known as alkaloids if they contain nitrogen) were isolated by chemists at that time. It then became possible for the pharmacologist to study the actions of the pure substance on animals and animal tissues. These actions, or some of them, could be related to the *mode of action* of this drug in the treatment of disease.

The next step was for the chemist to determine the complete molecular configuration of these agents, often a difficult task as their structures can be incredibly complex. The way in which the atoms of carbon, hydrogen, oxygen and nitrogen are arranged in morphine, for example, was suggested in 1925, but confirmed only as recently as 1952. Confirmation of a proposed structure requires the complete building up of the compound from simpler substances using unambiguous chemical reactions and pathways. This building up is known as chemical synthesis.

Once the structure of an active drug is known with certainty, some important possibilities arise. The fact that the drug can now be synthesized in the laboratory means that it is no longer necessary to grow the herb, extract the drug and purify it. However, in some cases it may be more economical to let the plant perform the synthesis. This is true of morphine even today; laboratory synthesis would be too expensive and time-consuming.

Next, pharmacological studies may identify active groups within the drug molecule. This has led to the concept of structure-activity relationship, in which the activity of the drug is attributed to certain specific arrangements of the atoms in the molecule. If it seems that large parts of the molecule of the natural substance play no vital role in its characteristic actions, it may be possible to synthesize a simpler molecule containing only the active groups. The simpler compound, or analogue, may not only be cheaper to manufacture but also possess fewer of the toxic or other undesirable properties of the plant drug (though there is no guarantee of this).

Studies of this kind have led to the discovery of many analogues of natural drugs, e.g., meperidine, fentanyl and methadone which have actions similar to morphine, but are easier to make in the laboratory. They have some advantages over morphine in medical treatment, e.g., fentanyl is eighty times more potent than morphine, depresses respiration less and is active for a shorter time; all can be taken orally. Pancuronium is a synthetic muscle relaxant used in surgery similar in chemical structure to natural curare. But these drugs have their drawbacks too.

The natural substance itself may be submitted to chemical manipulations in order to improve its efficacy, and perhaps also to reduce its toxicity. Such derivatives of the plant drug can be described as semi-synthetic. The basic core of the penicillin molecule has been modified to produce a family of semi-synthetic penicillins with specially useful actions on bacterial infections. Morphine can be treated with acetic anhydride to form diacetylmorphine or heroin. This derivative was originally applied enthusiastically to the cure of morphine addiction, on the grounds that the addicts gave up their morphine when offered heroin! It soon became clear that heroin was not only a better pain-killer (analgesic) than morphine, but more dangerously addictive as well.

There is no limit to the number of new compounds that the organic chemist can synthesize, and many of these unnatural substances have turned out to possess useful therapeutic properties. In fact, it has to be admitted that more therapeutic successes have been the result of chance synthesis than of logical considerations based on structure-activity relationship. This, of course, is a reflection of our relative ignorance, even today, of the exact ways in which drug molecules interact with the body's cellular machinery. However, computers are now beginning to help pharmacologists to study in three-dimensional detail the structural interactions between a drug and the cellular components on which it acts. This should greatly improve the logical design of new drugs based on structure-activity relationship. The technique is known as computer-aided drug design (CADD)[1] (see Preface, p. x).

During the twentieth century, the synthesis of new drugs has been largely taken over by the big pharmaceutical firms, which developed as offshoots from the chemical and dyestuffs industries, e.g., Imperial Chemical Industries (ICI), IG Farbenindustrie and others. These pharmaceutical firms have expert chemists and well-organized facilities for testing their new compounds for pharmacological activity. Much capital is invested in these researches which are carried out on a massive scale. In 1958, for example, 114,600 new chemicals were synthesized and tested by drug firms throughout the world. However, only about 44 of these (0.04%) were regarded as useful enough to be marketed as drugs for medical treatment. Even this low success rate can ensure considerable profits for these firms, and, of course, profit is the major incentive for the vast amount of capital and work involved.

The impact of the pharmaceutical industry on medical practice has grown explosively over the past fifty to sixty years. In 1935, Gerhard

Domagk (1895–1964), working for the IG Farbendustrie in Germany, discovered Prontosil, the parent compound of the sulphonamide group of antibacterial agents. Penicillin was first isolated at Oxford University, England, in 1941, but its production on a commercial scale required the capital and facilities of the American pharmaceutical industry. The development of the semi-synthetic penicillin analogues was achieved wholly by the drug firms, and since the World War II they have enormously increased the range and efficacy of drugs in all other categories.

This drug explosion has contributed immeasurably to the increased effectiveness of medical treatment, but it does create an added burden for the practising doctor who has to be familiar with the way through what some have called the therapeutic jungle. He has to be aware that the flood of new preparations coming onto the market may carry dangerous and often unsuspected toxicities, precisely because they are in general more effective in the treatment of disease.

For this reason, to ensure that the present-day physician is competent to guide his patients safely through the therapeutic jungle, he has to be taught as a medical student about the ways drugs act in the body, the exact indications for their use and their possible dangers. This education has to be continued throughout his professional life with regular refresher courses and other measures. A relatively new type of specialist, the clinical pharmacologist, can play a vital role in this process. A clinical pharmacologist is someone well versed in the basic mechanisms of drug action, as well as being an experienced physician in his own right. All reputable schools of medicine today have departments of clinical pharmacology to coordinate basic teaching about drugs with the regular course in applied pharmacology and therapeutics. Such departments can also make an important contribution to continuing education for practising physicians, especially in the field of pharmacokinetics (see Chap. 12, p. 83).

In spite of this, the training of doctors in the well-informed use of modern synthetic drugs often leaves much to be desired. Wrong prescribing, or the prescribing of too many drugs (polypharmacy), especially in older patients, can cause serious, even fatal, reactions. These unfortunate outcomes, often publicized in the press, have led to a renewed faith in the virtues of herbal medicine in some circles. The herbal enthusiasts are still with us and retain an irrational feeling that biologically-made agents are innately superior to man-made ones in the treatment of disease. Both, however, are chemical compounds and exert their pharmacological and therapeutic effects by precisely the same mechanisms. All that we have said about synthetic drugs applies equally to substances extracted from plants. Comments not infrequently seen in the press that some new herbal preparation being investigated in the laboratory will be free of side effects, just because it is of herbal origin, should be regarded with scepticism. For example, the Guy's Hospital Toxicology Unit in London sees three to five cases of liver failure per month caused by herbal remedies![2]

If herbal extracts or preparations do sometimes seem less toxic than synthetic drugs, it is usually due to their possessing a low concentration of active principle, which, of course, is liable to make them less potent. Herbal medicines are often more pleasant to take. They may be adequate for mild and self-limiting illnesses, and the well-known placebo effect is not to be despised in such cases. For serious disease, however, they tend to give little relief. We cannot turn back the clock, nor would it be desirable to do so. Modern synthetic drugs have revolutionized, and will continue to revolutionize the medical treatment of disease. Their dangers, though real, can be minimized if rightly used by doctors rigorously trained in the science of drug action, and kept up-to-date by the clinical pharmacologists.

3

What's Your Poison?

Man has an inborn craving for medicine ...
The desire to take medicine is one feature
which distinguishes man, the animal,
from his fellow creatures.

Sir William Osler (1894)

The craving for some kind of medication, referred to by the famous Victorian physician Sir William Osler, is being indulged in today more than ever before in the long history of mankind. We owe this to the ingenuity of the pharmacologist, the growth of the pharmaceutical industry and the wider availability of medical care.

A textbook of therapeutics published in 1980[1] reported that in Britain, on average, every member of the population consulted his doctor three times a year and received a prescription for 1.6 items at two of these consultations. Since many people do not need to see a doctor in any given year, obviously a sizeable minority spent much of their time in the doctor's office and consumed a large and varied menu of drugs. It is likely to be much the same today.

A survey of an Australian town of 15,700 inhabitants revealed that over a period of two weeks, only 11% reported neither illness nor drug ingestion. 66% had taken some medication, and 50% of this group took more than one drug preparation. Amazingly, about 60% of the preparations were self-prescribed, and only 40% were prescribed by doctors (or, in a few cases, pharmacists). Presumably 23% regarded themselves as ill, but did not seek or require drug treatment.

In the USA, during 1996, the average physician is said to have written

12,000 prescriptions for a national total of about 2.4 billion. (These figures sound almost impossible!) 2.5 million of these were for children under eighteen. The drug industry spent $12.5 billion promoting these medications, and the cost to the consumer was $85 billion. It has been suggested (cynically?) that only half of these produced the desired therapeutic result. The US drug industry also spent $2.5 billion on advertising its over-the-counter (OTC) drugs, and in view of this, it is not surprising that consumers bought $20 billion worth of these products.

The use of chemical substances to relieve the stress and anxiety of modern life is notoriously widespread. Many of these anti-anxiety (anxiolytic) drugs are benzodiazepine derivatives, i.e., chemical modifications of a basic benzodiazepine structure. More than 2,000 benzodiazepines have been synthesized in the laboratory, but of these only a handful (ten to twelve in the USA) are available for treating anxiety or insomnia. A 1988 report in the *British Medical Journal* claims that anxiolytics are taken daily for twelve months or longer by 3.1% of the British population. The corresponding figures for the USA and Europe are 1.8 and 1.6 respectively. Occasional use of benzodiazepines is, of course, much commoner; in 1986 it was estimated that an average of one out of ten adult Americans swallows benzodiazepines during the course of a year. Since 1973, these agents have been known to possess definite abuse potential, and though there has been some decrease in use in recent years, they are, nevertheless, still widely prescribed by the medical profession.

In spite of the lower figures (1.6%) for Europe, it seems that the French are virtually the world record-holders in the use of anxiolytics and sleeping pills, according to a 1991 article in the newspaper *Le Monde* entitled "A Nation of Hypochondriacs?" This is not only true of anxiolytics; the French consume fifty packets of drugs per head per year, twice as many as the Germans and three times as many as the Americans. One of the major causes of France's very high drug consumption is the attitude of their doctors who feel a compulsion to prescribe a drug (or several drugs) after every consultation.

These figures indicate that, as might be expected, there are national and cultural differences in drug-taking patterns, and in medical treatment in general. The American medical journalist Lynn Payer[2] has investigated some of these in a book published in 1988. Suppositories, rather than oral agents, for minor ailments such as headaches are popular in France, Germany and Austria. German doctors regard low blood pressure as a disorder that requires vigorous treatment with one or more of the 85 available preparations. Such a symptom in the USA would merely entitle the patient to lower life insurance premiums. French medicine concentrates (not unreasonably) on strengthening the *terrain* (roughly translated: constitution or resistance) of the individual, so that he can more readily repulse the noxious invader, hence the emphasis on tonics and vitamins, smaller doses of potent drugs and a reluctance to resort to antibiotics. German romanticism (according to Payer) leads to an obsession with the heart, and Germans use about six times the quantity of heart drugs than the French or British, though there is no evidence that heart disease is more common in Germany. British medicine is coolly pragmatic, reluctant to accept new treatments without the backing of strictly controlled random clinical trials, and conservative with surgery and grueling drug régimes like cancer chemotherapy.

Everywhere, probably, the elderly are more likely to be taking medication than the young; 11% of Americans over 65 in 1980 received 30% of all drugs prescribed medically. Since older people are in general more sensitive to drugs, this can lead to unexpected toxicities. In fact, it is estimated that 73,000 senior Americans died in 1987 from taking the wrong drug, from improper dosage of the right drug, or from fatal drug reactions and interactions. This figure exceeds the total of 58,000 servicemen killed during the Vietnam War. Indeed, 73,000 may be an underestimate since there is an understandable tendency on death certificates to record the disease under treatment as cause of death, and few autopsies are performed in such cases.

Elderly patients may suffer from more than one disease, and so are more likely to be given several drugs at the same time (so-called polypharmacy; see p. 54). This means the greater danger of adverse interactions; 40% of those with such reactions are over sixty. Roughly 30% of older patients use eight or more medications simultaneously, and those over 75 receive an average of seventeen different prescriptions each year.

Apart from prescription drugs, pharmacies and drug stores offer a glittering display of well-advertized over-the-counter (OTC) preparations. The 1991 figures show that an amazing 20% of drug expenditure in West Germany goes to medicines not prescribed by physicians. A 1972 UK survey revealed that 99% of a sample of family homes contained well-stocked medicine cabinets. Of the average of 10.3 items per cabinet, three were prescription drugs and 7.7 were OTC preparations. Some of the most common of the latter were analgesics (e.g., aspirin), skin creams, liniments, cough lozenges, and eye, ear and nose drops. In general, preparations for self-administration are designed to provide short-term relief of mild symptoms where accurate diagnosis of their cause is not required, and where the margin of safety of the drug components is wide. Nevertheless, patients should be advised to inform their physician of any OTC preparations they are taking, in case of possible interactions of a prescription drug with one or more of the OTC drugs (see Chap. 7, p. 55).

In spite of the obvious popularity of drug ingestion among the public, the average man or woman in the street has little knowledge about what happens to these drugs in his or her body or how they act. He or she is hardly aware of their possible hazards; and there seems no great attempt to educate the layman in these matters by the medical profession. In fact, as already mentioned (p. 23), there are doctors who do not adequately inform their patients about the drugs they prescribe, because their own education in this field has been sadly deficient. There was in the past, undoubtedly, a gross under-evaluation of the importance of the study of drug action in the curricula of many medical schools throughout the world. Such schools produced graduates who, in their practices, became easy prey for the not entirely disinterested blandishments of the *detail men* from the drug firms. Even today, the influence of the pharmaceutical industry with its lavish advertizing, and not always completely honest promotional activities, may seduce the medical profession into the unwise over-prescribing of the plethora of potent drugs available on the market (see Chap. 9 for a fuller discussion).

Behind all this is the *craving for medicine* mentioned by Osler. Even in prehistoric times primitive man could indulge that craving with the herbal concoctions provided by the medicine man. The strange thing is that the medicine man must often have cured his patients. His theories of disease may have been false, but his drugs, though limited in number, were sometimes moderately active and he was no doubt expert in their practical use. There are some other reasons for his therapeutic successes, which are instructive to consider, even today.

First of all, many diseases are self-curing, or at least self-limiting, so that even inactive drugs may appear to effect a cure. The common cold is said to persist for two weeks with drug treatment, fourteen days with no drug treatment. The modern physician, like his ancestor the medicine man, is not averse to taking credit for *curing* an illness which was really dealt with by the body's *vis medicatrix naturae* (natural healing force). Over-enthusiastic reports of new therapeutic discoveries, especially for diseases of an intermittent kind (e.g., multiple sclerosis), appear frequently in the press, and raise false hopes which are later cruelly betrayed.

Another important reason for some of the successes of traditional medicine is the existence of the *placebo effect* (Placebo is Latin for "I will please"). It is well known that a drug given by a man of authority and confidence to a sick and suggestible individual, who desperately wants to be cured, may have a therapeutic effect above and beyond that to be expected on a strictly pharmacological basis. In fact, the drug can be virtually inert, and yet be remarkably effective in certain vague illnesses like headaches, which often have a considerable psychological element in their causation. Also, certain patients show this placebo effect to an exaggerated degree, and are known as placebo reactors.

Even the modern scientifically-trained doctor in his white coat has this aura of authority which can stimulate the placebo effect, especially when he is enthusiastically trying out a new drug. This is no doubt the basis of the cynical remark of some physicians: *"Use a new drug while it still works!"*, i.e., while doctors and patients still have faith in it. Of course, in the absence of a really effective drug for a particular disease, there is no reason why a doctor should not intentionally exploit the placebo effect for the benefit of the patient. But in testing new drugs, it is essential to eliminate the placebo effect by careful design of the clinical trials, in order to arrive at an unbiased assessment of its alleged superiority over existing agents (see Chap. 4, p. 32).

Taking drugs for even the most trivial of illnesses is not the only form in which Osler's *inborn craving* reveals itself. There is the age-old need to escape from the dullness or the agony of daily living by the ingestion or injection of chemicals, which alter mind and consciousness. Since such drugs are almost always self-administered, leading often to dependency and severe addiction, the social and personal problems engendered by them are enormous (see Part II). We must not forget, too, that some chemicals are absorbed inadvertently and often unknowingly by large populations in our increasingly technological world; these are the poisons of industrial origin (Chap. 15, p. 103).

Whatever the source of these poisons, and whether they are ingested intentionally or not, it has become mandatory in the modern world to test these agents for their effects on human health. Some ways in which this is done will now be described.

4

Trying It on the Dog

A pharmacologist speaking to the American Medical Association in 1929 said: "Many drug firms make the mistake of believing that their chemists can furnish trustworthy pharmacological opinion … There is no short cut from chemical laboratory to clinic except one that passes *too close to the morgue*."[1] This solemn warning refers not only to substances that are intended for use in treating disease, but to any agent applied, or gaining access, to the human organism, e.g., food or drug additives (colours, flavours, sweeteners, solvents, preservatives), cosmetics, and pesticides. A tragic example of ignoring this possible danger occurred only eight years later (1937) in the US when diethylene glycol was used as solvent for the newly discovered drug sulphanilamide.[2] The drug itself was effective and relatively non-toxic, but the solvent caused the deaths of 105 patients, an outcome which could have been avoided if it had first been tested for lethal actions in small animals.

The pharmaceutical industry, in fact industry in general, has taken these lessons to heart, especially since the thalidomide disaster of 1960–61. Any new chemical compound that is likely to be absorbed in some way or other, or used for some purpose or other, by the human organism must be carefully screened for possible toxicity before it is marketed. This, however, is not quite as simple as it might seem. Let us consider the problem with new drugs.

Initially, screening tests for a new drug are carried out on healthy live animals, or on organs or tissues from recently killed animals. If the new drug is a simple modification of an old drug with known actions, then the chief aim will be to compare relative potencies for these particular actions. These actions, of course, could be either therapeutic or toxic in nature.

A completely novel compound of unknown potentialities is, however, more likely to be submitted to *random screening*, using a whole battery of tests on different animals. The results of these tests are evaluated and recorded, and provide a so-called *profile* of pharmacological activity for that compound. Any chemical which shows promise is put through further careful testing, again on live animals or on isolated tissues. The commonest animal species employed for this purpose are mice, rats, cats, dogs, guinea-pigs, hamsters, rabbits and monkeys.

A special refinement is to test the new drugs on a disease induced in animals. This may provide useful information about those diseases, e.g., infections or cancer, which can be more or less precisely duplicated in an animal species. Unfortunately, much human disease cannot be exactly copied in animals, and we have to make do with a *model* that often bears only a superficial relationship to the real thing. For example, a kind of rat can be bred which becomes spontaneously hypertensive, (i.e., its blood pressure rises above normal), and this can be used to test drugs for the treatment of hypertension in man. However, the causes of hypertension in man are varied, possibly different from those in the experimental rat, or even quite unknown. Drugs effective for rat hypertension may prove a disappointment in man. Furthermore, for many human diseases there is still not even an approximate animal model.

At this stage, those involved in testing drugs must remember that chemicals are poisons, and an effective drug will be no use if it is dangerously toxic to patients. Again, animals remain, at least for the time being, our first line of defence. So-called *acute toxicity* tests determine the adverse effects of a single dose in animals, and particularly the approximate dose which will cause death.

For statistical reasons it would be inaccurate and possibly very misleading to measure the dose of a substance which kills an animal, or even the dose which kills all of the animals in a group. If groups of animals are given increasing doses of a chemical, beginning with small doses, and the percentage of animals dying in each group is observed, one obtains what is known as a dose-response curve. The typical curve is said to be S-shaped (sigmoid), but is actually a distorted S with almost horizontal lower and upper sections joined by a forward-leaning and rising curve. Small doses produce no deaths (lower horizontal), large doses above a certain level produce 100% mortality (upper horizontal), and in between the rising portion of the S-curve shows mortality increasing from 0–100% as the dose of the compound increases. Statistically, it is around the level of 50% mortality that the rate of change of lethality with dose is greatest, and this is the most sensitive part of the curve to work with to obtain accurate and informative measurements of the toxicity of a chemical. Hence it is customary to measure a dose which will kill, on average, half (50%) of a group, and this is known as the Lethal Dose Fifty (LD_{50}) of the drug for that particular species of animal. Because of the variability of response inherent in all biological systems, the accuracy of the estimate of the LD_{50} will also depend on the number of animals used. Increasing the size of the group will give a statistically more reliable figure.[3]

We can also measure, in the same animal species and using the same route of administration, the dose of the drug which will produce the desired therapeutic effect in 50% of a group. If we call this the Effective Dose Fifty (ED_{50}), we can calculate the ratio LD_{50}/ED_{50} for that drug in that animal. This ratio is known as the Therapeutic Index (TI).

It should not be difficult to convince the reader that a possible new drug with a TI of less than one had better remain on the laboratory shelf, or, perhaps, be exploited as a miracle rat poison.

Clearly, the TI of a drug should be greater than, and preferably much greater than, unity, i.e., there should be a wide margin of safety between the curative and lethal doses, especially in humans. With penicillin, a natural product, the TI is very large indeed (except in the occasional subject hypersensitive to it). The TI of digoxin, another natural substance isolated from the foxglove leaf, is only about three. Here the margin of safety is small, and doses only a little above those necessary for a good therapeutic effect are liable to provide undesirable sublethal actions. For this reason, the physician finds digoxin a troublesome drug to administer safely *and* effectively. Incidentally, the TI of that element vital to life, oxygen, is also about three![4] Penicillin, digoxin and oxygen are cited as contrasting examples in order to underline the fact that natural origin is no guarantee of lack of toxicity.

Apart from acute toxicity (causing immediate death), it is essential to look for the subacute and chronic toxicities of a new drug. These are determined by exposing animals to various doses of the substance continuously over periods from one week to the lifetime of the species tested. This kind of test is especially important for those drugs which are going to be administered to patients for long periods. The toxic effects most feared are: those on the bone marrow causing blood disorders; impairment of reproductive function; teratogenesis (production of a deformed foetus); and oncogenesis (production of malignant tumours).

The food intake, growth, general health, activity and reproductive ability are monitored in the groups of animals under observation. Urine and blood are examined for adverse changes, and from time to time a few animals from the group are killed (*sacrificed,* in toxicological jargon) so that organs and tissues can be looked at for evidence of damage.

The sacrifice of large numbers of animals to check the pharmacological activities, and the acute and chronic toxicities, of new chemicals is distasteful to many laymen, and causes some misgivings in scientific circles. Should we do something about this, and if so, what? Before discussing this question, it is interesting to outline briefly the history of how animals came to be employed in scientific research.

A compassionate concern for the welfare of animals, both wild and domesticated, has probably never been an outstanding characteristic of *Homo sapiens* until quite recent times. The study of *lower* forms of life as models to throw light on the anatomy and physiology of the human organism began seriously only in the early and middle decades of the nineteenth century. Presumably this attitude was influenced by a growing awareness of man's animal ancestry based on the theories of evolution developing at that time. Such researches on animals were enthusiastically carried out first in France and Germany, but did not become acceptable in Great Britain until around 1870, after the discovery of anaesthesia. It was then possible to perform surgical experiments on animals without inflicting too much pain. Animal studies have aided our understanding of many of the physiological and biochemical processes occurring in the human body, and the knowledge obtained in this way has contributed immeasurably to advances in medical science over the past hundred years or so.

Pharmacologists, in particular, found animals to be invaluable for revealing the biological properties of chemical substances, and, once pure compounds were extracted from natural sources, they could determine the actual dose required to produce a certain pharmacological effect. Equally, they could determine the doses that were toxic to the animal. They then devised, by an ingenious reversal of principle, an original way of using animals to measure the quantity of a pharmacologically active substance in an impure extract. This process was known as biological assay (or bioassay). Some biological activity of the substance being investigated in the extract, e.g., contraction of a piece of isolated guinea-pig ileum, or the rate of beating of an isolated rabbit heart, is converted instrumentally into a quantitative measurement, and compared with the activity of a standard solution of the pure substance. Such methods are obligatory if the active substance cannot be quantified by any existing chemical reaction, or (as is often the case) the amounts present are too minute to be measured by chemical reactions. They are (or were) specially valuable in following the purification of a new active substance.

The rapid growth of experimental pharmacology in the early years of the last century depended enormously on the use of animals in studying the actions, and measuring the amounts present in extracts, of such physiologically important substances as acetylchlorine, adrenaline, histamine and others. Even the isolation of the enkephalins (the pain-suppressing agents in the brain), which was achieved as recently as 1975, was monitored by observing their actions on guinea-pig or mouse tissues (see Chap. 20, p. 142). Many drugs used in therapeutics were discovered to depend for their efficacy on some kind of interference with the physiological actions of these naturally occurring agents. Moreover, industry was legally required to utilize bioassay techniques to standardize certain commercial preparations for which there was no suitable chemical or physicochemical method, e.g., digoxin in digitalis extracts, insulin in pig or beef pancreatic extracts.

The use of animals in academic research grew rapidly after the mid-nineteenth century and into the twentieth century, but in recent years it has been levelling off or even falling. One of a number of reasons for this is the development of much more sensitive methods of a physico-chemical nature for measuring low concentrations of physiologically active substances. Bioassay would nowadays be regarded as an outmoded procedure in most laboratories. As a matter of fact, the majority of animal experiments today are carried out by industry. The pharmaceutical firms, in particular, do the bulk of the work outlined at the beginning of this chapter: the testing of new compounds for therapeutic activity and for toxicity. Chemical firms, too, are bound by government regulatory bodies to submit all new chemicals to stringent tests before they can be made generally available to the public for agricultural, domestic and other purposes. It has not been possible so far to obviate the use of animals (so-called *in vivo* testing) in these necessary screening processes, and substitute *in vitro* tests, in spite of the efforts of scientists and animal welfare advocates. This brings us to a brief discussion of those movements, often highly emotional and irrational, which seek to abolish totally the use of animals in all scientific and medical research and in industry.

Anti-vivisectionists have always been very active in the UK. When animals began to be used there in 1870 after the introduction of general anaesthesia, there was much debate about whether the procedures were ethically justifiable. A Royal Commission was appointed in 1875 and led to the passing of the Cruelty to Animals Act in 1876, which closely regulated scientific experiments on animals. Some legislators wanted to ban completely all experiments with cats, dogs and equidae (horses, donkeys, mules), but eventually these *were* allowed under special certificates. This Act is still in force in the UK, which has probably the most stringently regulated and inspected system of animal experimentation in the world. Moreover, further animal protection legislation was passed in 1986, the Animals (Scientific Procedures) Act. The UK together with the European Economic Community has recommended the abolition of the LD_{50} test and its replacement by a *fixed dose procedure* using fewer animals and causing less pain and distress (1990). In spite of this, or perhaps as part of it, anti-vivisection sentiment continues to flourish, becoming particularly active in the 1930s and the 1980s. Sir Andrew Huxley, in his foreword to Professor W.D.M. Paton's book, *Man and Mouse: Animals in Medical Research*[5] (1994), wrote: "We are now in the midst of another wave, in which terrorist groups break into laboratories and use letter-bombs to intimidate those who dare to remind the public of the advances in curative medicine and in public health that have followed from experiments on living animals."

The tendentious and misleading propaganda put out by these extremist organizations, with appealing photographs of dogs or cats, omits to mention that in the UK, 80% of all animal experiments are performed on less appealing rats and mice. Dogs and cats are involved in only 0.47% of the total. The layman is easily confused today by this adverse publicity in a world in which medical research has expanded enormously, and become mostly too esoteric for all but the professional biologist to comprehend. Paton, formerly Professor of Pharmacology at Oxford University, points out that if animal experimentation is wrong now, it was wrong 100 years ago, and then proposes a test of *deletion* whereby the effects of abolishing animal research today is predicted by considering the effects of a similar abolition in the past. We might not, for example, have typhoid vaccine (ca. 1894), polio vaccine (ca. 1958), streptomycin for tuberculosis (early 1940s), local anaesthetics (ca. 1902), insulin (1921–22), or leukemia and cancer chemotherapy (ca. 1950). The development of all these agents, and many others, required either direct experiments with animals, or was based on the body of physiological and biochemical knowledge obtained in that way. He trenchantly concludes his book with these words: " ... animal hooligans, mostly of the healthiest generation this country [Britain] has ever seen because of past medical research ... harass the experimenters, the animal breeders, and the industry ... Animal experimentation is essential in medical and veterinary research. Those who unreasonably harass and restrict it now will carry a grave responsibility for the unnecessary ignorance and unnecessary suffering that will result in the future."[6]

There are, of course, moderate animal welfare groups whose main concern is to seek reasonable alternatives to the use of animals in research, and these are supported by responsible scientists, if only on economic grounds. Suitable healthy animals for research are expensive nowadays, and to obtain adequate supplies of the necessary pure strains of a species (to minimize biological variations in response) demands properly controlled breeding facilities. Organizations such as FRAME (Fund for Replacement of Animals in Medical Experiments) started in the UK in 1978, AFAAR (American Fund for Alternatives to Animals in Research in 1978, and IFER (International Foundation for Ethical Research, USA) in 1987. They are specially interested in developing new *in vitro* methods of toxicity testing. *In vitro* testing avoids using intact higher animals by working with bacteria, cultured animal cells, fertilized chicken eggs and frog embryos. In time, it may be possible to test chemicals on cultures of human cells from various organs and tissues; this would provide direct information about a chemical's toxicity in humans. However, though progress toward these ends is being slowly made, in the battle for drug safety some use of whole animals is likely to be unavoidable for many years to come.[7]

Apart from ethical objections, it has to be realized that animals experiments also have serious scientific limitations and pitfalls. Different species of animal, and even different strains of the same species, may react differently to the same drug, and there is no guarantee that findings in animals necessarily apply to man. In other words, a drug that appears to be effective and harmless in animals may be useless in man because of unexpected and unacceptable toxicity. Conversely, a drug discarded because of high toxicity in animals *might* have proved miraculously therapeutic in man. But who would have dared to try it?

The phenomenon of *species difference*, which is often based on variations in the tissue enzymes acting on the drug, bedevils all testing of drugs on animals, and there are no simple solutions to the problems it poses. This fact, but not its explanation, was quite clearly recognized by those suspicious and unpopular medieval princes who employed human food tasters in their banquet halls, rather than flinging samples of the fare to their dogs.

Nevertheless, careful preliminary tests on animals remain the necessary protective hurdle that a drug must clear before it is administered at all to man. The occasional disasters which have occurred since that warning to the American Medical Association in 1929 can sometimes be attributed to ignorance and carelessness on the part of the drug firm concerned, but not always and rather rarely today. Whatever the cause of these disasters and the public scandals they often lead to, the trend since 1929 has been for government agencies increasingly to regulate the manufacture, testing and marketing of new drugs, especially in the USA and the UK.

Today it may take around ten years and cost about 100 million dollars to bring a new drug to the market in the US. Controls by the Food and Drug Administration (FDA) are now so strict and time-consuming that new drugs of undoubted value may come onto the market several years after their widespread medical use in other countries. It is a moot question whether these bureaucratic delays have, on balance, prevented more suffering by blocking an unexpectedly toxic drug than they have caused by depriving seriously ill patients of a valuable new remedy. Certainly, in the case of the thalidomide catastrophe of 1960–61, the US public was saved from tragedy by the leaden hand of governmental interference.

The teratogenic effects of the hypnotic drug thalidomide on the foetus, and the subsequent birth of infants with phocomelia or *seal extremities*, has had an understandably powerful emotional impact on the public's attitude to the dangers of drugs. The shadow of this heart-rending disaster still hangs over the medical profession and the pharmaceutical industry. The industry, in particular, has been put on the defensive, and is now quick to avoid bad publicity (and falling share prices) by withdrawing any new drug that is linked, rightly or wrongly, to the appearance of adverse effects in patients.

We now know that the teratogenic effects of thalidomide are due to a metabolite of the drug which is formed only in certain species. The metabolite is formed in rabbits, but not in rats, and unfortunately rats were used to test the actions of thalidomide in pregnancy, as was customary at the time. The firm that promoted this drug was just plain unlucky; any other firm would equally have failed to reveal this dire toxicity. It was clinical reports in the UK of thalidomide causing peripheral neuritis (not an unusual nor specially dangerous side effect) which triggered a merciful pause in the routine administrative machinery of governmental approval in the US. During the delay, the more serious toxicity came to light elsewhere.

The attempts, after the disaster in Europe, to suppress information in the press, and the interminable legal wrangling over reasonable compensation to the victims, however, make a less savoury story. In fact, who should bear the responsibility when a widely used drug reveals unsuspected and serious toxicity, and what compensation should be paid to the victims and by whom, are difficult questions that provide a field day for lawyers. We shall return to this problem later (Chap. 7, p. 56), but first we must describe more fully some of the clinical tests on human subjects which a new drug has to undergo before it can be finally released to the medical profession.

5

The Proof of the Pudding ...

Medical treatment is an art founded on
conjecture and improved by murder.

Sir Anthony Carlisle

After the exhaustive studies on animals outlined in the last chapter, the
cautious administration of a new drug to man (or woman) can be
undertaken with reasonable confidence that at least no immediate disaster
will occur. It would no longer be quite fair to echo Sir Anthony Carlisle, an
early nineteenth century therapeutic nihilist, whose cynicism was no doubt
justified at that time.

In the US, where these matters are claimed to be more strictly
regulated than elsewhere, it is at the outset of human testing that the Food
and Drug Administration (FDA) enters the picture. The drug sponsor,
normally a commercial firm, must outline the various trials proposed on
healthy volunteers and on patients, and wait for a month or so while the
FDA makes sure that no unwarranted risks are being run (FDA Thirty-day
Safety Review). If the FDA is satisfied that protocols of the animal studies
indicate that the drug should be reasonably safe in man, it is made an
"investigational new drug" (IND) and approved for clinical testing in
humans.

Tests on human subjects are divided into three phases. In Phase I,
increasing doses of the IND, starting at about one-tenth or less of the
expected effective dosage, are given to a small group of normal healthy
volunteers. This is to confirm that the substance does have the desired
pharmacological or therapeutic activity, and is not unexpectedly toxic. The
opportunity is also taken to study the distribution of the drug in the body,

its excretion and its metabolism (pharmacokinetics). This work is carried out largely by clinical pharmacologists.

In Phase II, clinical pharmacologists study the actions of the drug in a limited number of selected patients suffering from the disease which the agent is expected to cure or alleviate. The efficacy, the most suitable dosage scheme and the route of administration are evaluated, and, once more, any side effects are carefully looked for.

If Phase II shows promising results, practising clinicians now take over and plan an extensive series of clinical trials in a much larger number of patients. This is Phase III, in which the drug is used as it would be in medical practice. There are, however, some limitations to these procedures. Usually Phase III trials involve not more than 3,000 patients, and of these only a few hundred are treated for longer than three to six months, even if it is expected that the drug may need to be used for longer periods for optimal therapeutic effect. Clinical trials on children and pregnant women are, for obvious reasons, restricted. Clearly, certain adverse effects that may appear when the drug is accepted for wider application could well be missed at this stage. Nevertheless, if Phase III is regarded as confirming effectiveness and safety, the sponsor next applies to the FDA for approval to market the drug ("new drug application" or NDA). Phases I-III may take two to ten years, with an average of five to six years. The FDA review itself may take from two months to seven years (average 2.6 years), and is carried out by a committee composed of physicians, pharmacists, chemists, pharmacologists and other experts.

A similar process has existed for many years in Britain under the auspices of the Committee on Safety of Medicines. This is now being integrated with a comparable EU (European Union) organization.

Obviously, in the USA a new drug has to clear many hurdles before the FDA permits its general use by the medical profession. Even then, control is not relaxed, nor should it be. Because of the limitations of the Phase III testing, the drug manufacturer must report to the FDA at regular intervals any problems in production, or the appearance of unexpected toxicities during clinical use. Moreover, physicians using the drug are encouraged to inform the manufacturer or the FDA of any adverse effects seen during their clinical practice.

The aims and procedures of the clinical trials carried out during Phase III require further explanation. It is realized today that sound statistical planning of these trials is necessary, since dependence on the uncontrolled clinical impressions of biassed observers could be misleading. A therapeutic trial has been defined as "a carefully and ethically designed experiment aimed to answer some precisely framed question. In its most rigorous form it demands equivalent groups of patients concurrently treated in different ways. These groups are constructed by the random allocation of patients to one or other treatments."[1]

The use of equivalent groups of patients and different treatments is essential to provide a sound basis for comparison, but even this precaution does not go quite far enough if one wishes to eliminate the placebo effect. If the physician and the patients know who is getting the new drug, the enthusiasm of the doctors and nurses and the hopes and anxieties of the patients create a fertile soil for possible bias due to a placebo reaction.

A reputable way to avoid such a bias is to use a double-blind technique. (This can lead to bad jokes about the double-blind leading the double-blind!) The new drug, and the other treatment for comparison (which may be a dummy tablet of identical appearance, or an older established drug), are given in such a way that the subject (the first blind man) does not know which he is receiving. The physician-investigator (the second blind man) is also unaware which treatment is which. The treatment code is held by an outsider, e.g., the hospital pharmacist, and is usually broken only at the end of the trial when the results are evaluated.

Although the idea of experimenting on sick patients may seem soulless to some people, it must be recognized that, without randomized controlled clinical trials of the kind described above, progress in therapeutics would grind to a halt. Any doctor giving any drug to any patient is, in a sense, carrying out a unique experiment, since no patient is exactly similar to another. The doctor must always be on the alert for an unexpected outcome of treatment, and particularly for the appearance of adverse effects.

Occasionally, of course, the findings of a clinical trial may quickly turn out to be more favourable to a new drug than expected, revealing it as considerably more effective than the placebo and minimally toxic. In such cases, it would be unethical to continue treating sick patients with an inert placebo, and the trial should be discontinued. This situation occurred during clinical trials of the anti-breast cancer drug tamoxifen.

In the past, drug therapy was largely a matter of tradition or fashion. Positively harmful treatments remained in vogue for years, protected from criticism by the authority of a famous name. Since every drug administration is an experiment, it is obviously better to apply controlled statistical planning right from the start. In this way, the most effective (or the least ineffective) treatment can be revealed in the shortest possible time, with a saving of lives and money.

Nevertheless, ethical problems do arise in human drug trials, and in many parts of the world any research programme has to be submitted for approval to some kind of ethical review committee. One aspect, which can lead to difficulties, is the question of informed patient consent. The US FDA is against any patient being included in a Phase I or Phase II trial of an IND without his written consent, and a full explanation of the possible hazards involved. In Phase III, however, too much explanation could vitiate a strict double-blind procedure; but, at that stage, a new drug would have been tested sufficiently to make it unlikely that serious toxicity would be encountered.

Drug testing on so-called volunteers in prisons and other institutions has led to justifiable censure in the USA. The controlled diet, activity and environment in such places is helpful to investigators, but whether the inmates can really be said to have the freedom to give their uninfluenced consent to medical experimentation is a matter for some scepticism.

Today, an approved new drug in the hands of the medical practitioner will have been as meticulously tested as any product of modern industry. Yet it is, after all, a selective poison which must be prescribed with care and with attention to known and unknown toxicities. Some risk, however small, is inherent in drug therapy, and it is the responsibility of the well-trained physician to balance as conscientiously as he can the benefits against the dangers for the individual patient he plans to treat.

In severe and potentially fatal disease like cancer, effective drugs are, for reasons related to their mode of action, almost invariably highly toxic. The risks involved, however, are regarded as acceptable in the circumstances. In the milder forms of illness, especially where complete natural cure is to be expected, the acceptable risk must be very much lower. It has been suggested that a treatment may be taken as safe if the risk of serious toxicity falls below one in a hundred thousand.

This bare statistic is, of course, no comfort to that hundred thousandth patient (or his relatives), but we can put the situation into perspective by pointing out that in the UK every year, for example, there are at least about 6,000 fatal accidents in the home, 7,000 fatal vehicle accidents and 28,000 malignant lung cancers mostly related to cigarette smoking. On the other hand, only 40 to 50 times a year are drugs named on death certificates as the cause of death. Admittedly, drug fatalities may be somewhat underestimated since the patients concerned are usually seriously ill, and the doctor is liable to attribute death to the disease rather than to the drug. All the same, death from drug treatment is obviously a relatively minor risk in our dangerous modern world.

To ensure this degree of safety takes time. The period from initial testing to marketing approval may be ten years or longer, and this cannot all be attributed to bureaucratic procrastination. Such delays cause great concern to patients with life-threatening diseases like cancer, and especially to those with AIDS (acquired immune deficiency syndrome). AIDS is a new disease only recognized by the medical profession since 1982, and research to discover effective therapeutic agents is still in a more or less preliminary phase. Moreover, AIDS sufferers can die within two years of developing the full syndrome, and are naturally prepared to try any promising line of treatment. Some years ago the FDA was persuaded to relax standards for new drugs that showed some likelihood of at least prolonging life in these patients. Conditional approval for the early release of certain drugs was being given (1991) before they were fully tested, and even before their efficacy had been confidently established. This fast-track policy was not universally welcomed by physicians in view of the fact that existing drugs for AIDS are invariably, and possibly inevitably, very toxic and produce serious side effects. In fact, the FDA also promised to speed up the testing processes for all new drugs, but this turned out to be a retrograde step.

Certainly, it would seem that over the past few years the FDA has dangerously relaxed its criteria for approval of new drugs in all categories, leading to an increased number of hurried withdrawals prompted by unexpected reports of serious toxicities. As many as six drugs approved since 1993 were withdrawn on safety grounds in 1999 and 2000, two of these in the week of 19 March 2000.[2] One was cisapride (Propulsid), a drug widely promoted for heartburn that has been associated with heart rhythm abnormalities, leading to eight reports of death. Although the manufacturer (Janssen Pharmaceutica) stopped marketing cisapride in March 2000, the drug was permitted to remain on pharmacy shelves until mid-August 2000.[3] The other drug was the antidiabetic agent troglitazone (Rezulin); this caused severe liver and heart toxicity leading to a possible death toll of 26. Both drugs have been banned in the UK (troglitazone in December 1997), suggesting that the British Committee on Safety of Medicines is now more cautious in approving new drugs than the FDA.

All we have said so far applies, of course, to prescription drugs, and not to over-the-counter drugs which can be bought freely by the public at any pharmacy. These for obvious reasons tend to be rather non-potent drugs, useful only in minor disorders. Because of their low potency, they show correspondingly low toxicity, and the risk involved in reasonable self-medication can be accepted as negligible for all practical purposes. However, as will be mentioned later, occasional unpleasant reactions may occur if other, more potent, prescription drug are being given at the same time. Nor, until recently, have medical devices such as artificial joints or heart valves been submitted to rigorous clinical testing.

The prescription drug is a remarkable product of modern industry. Although it is marketed with known (and likely unknown) hazards for the benefit of the ultimate consumer, the patient, its sale is channelled through the medical practitioner whose primary responsibility is to decide whether the consumer should receive the drug. This is surely a unique state of affairs.

We rightly expect our automobiles, hair-dryers and other appliances to be 100% safe, and there is a public outcry if they are not. But we cannot expect our drugs to be 100% safe, by the very nature of their action; and, furthermore, the consumer, who is often seriously ill, is prepared to trade a reasonable risk against the promise of cure or relief.

Our drugs are checked and double-checked by the pharmaceutical industry, and administered with therapeutic expertise and constant vigilance to patients whose life might otherwise be short and miserable. At least, that is our hope and trust. Yet serious reactions to new drugs, which are inevitable from time to time, tend to get blown up out of all proportion by the media, and ascribed to negligence by the prescribing doctor and inadequate testing by the manufacturer.

I do not wish to canonize the drug industry whose advertizing and sales policies are not always above criticism, especially in the Third World countries. Nor, as pointed out above, is the FDA immune nowadays from criticism. Equally, I do not ignore the fact that there are doctors who use drugs incompetently. It is probably the doctor, the middleman between the manufacturer and the patient, who bears the greatest responsibility for the safe application of drugs; who must have the capability to assess from his knowledge of pharmacology and therapeutics the validity of the sometimes misleading or exaggerated claims made by the drug firms.

Even a fully approved and apparently safe new drug has to be carefully watched for many years after its release to the medical profession. The next two chapters will describe some of the problems that may arise during this most necessary period of vigilance.

6

Eternal Vigilance

Show me a safe drug, and I will show you
an ineffective drug!

Sir Derrick Dunlop

An adverse or toxic reaction to a drug has been defined[1] as "a harmful or
seriously unpleasant effect seen at doses intended to provide diagnosis,
prophylaxis or cure of a disease, which warrants reduction in dosage or
even complete withdrawal of the drug."

Sir Derrick, who was chairman from 1969 to 1971 of the UK
Committee on the Safety of Medicines, made a cogent, if slightly cynical,
observation. Certainly, important adverse reactions may not be recognized
until the drug has been in general medical use for a considerable period of
time. This fact need not be any reflection on the integrity of the drug
manufacturer, nor on the professional competence of the physician
prescribing the drug. Even drugs of venerable antiquity can turn up some
unpleasant surprises after decades of widespread administration. There is
no place for therapeutic complacency, and the price of safety is eternal
vigilance.

The mild analgesic phenacetin was first introduced in 1887, and it
became a popular constituent of widely used (and abused) over-the-counter
preparations for many years. It was only 66 years later that suspicion fell
on the drug as a possible cause, when taken habitually, of severe damage
to the kidneys (known as analgesic nephropathy). We are still not
absolutely sure of a direct cause-effect relationship in this case, and other
constituents of the analgesic mixtures may have been responsible, but the
circumstantial evidence was strong enough for most progressive

government health authorities to ban the sale of this drug to the general public. Since the ban, the incidence of analgesic nephropathy has declined except, for some unknown reason, in Australia.[2]

Aspirin, which must be one of the world's most widely used pain-killers, was first introduced into medicine in 1899 (see p. 196). Apart from its tendency in a few sensitive subjects to produce gastric irritation or even ulceration with blood loss and anaemia, it has always been regarded as one of the safest and most effective drugs in medicine. However, it has been realized only in recent years that children suffering from feverish illnesses due to a virus should not be given aspirin. In such cases the drug may cause Reye's Syndrome, a condition involving nausea, vomiting, lethargy, delirium and occasionally seizures with a 10–40% death rate.

Of course, if a drug commonly produces a *rare* disease or untoward effect, this will almost certainly have been picked up during clinical trials and before it is marketed. However, some special categories of patients, e. g., pregnant women, would never be asked to take part in clinical trials, and an uncommon result of administration in pregnancy would not be revealed at this stage. This is another contributory reason why the teratogenic activity of thalidomide was not discovered earlier. The wise physician nowadays is very reluctant to give any drug at all to a pregnant patient, especially during the first three months when the growing foetus is most sensitive to toxic agents.

The action of a drug which *commonly* induces a *common* side-effect may well remain undetected, because of the obvious difficulty of establishing a cause-effect relationship. Once suspicion is aroused, however, carefully planned statistical studies will confirm the correlation. A drug which *rarely* causes a *common* disorder is unlikely ever to be incriminated.

It is the drug that *rarely* provokes a *rare* toxicity or disorder in man which has caused the biggest problems, especially when the toxicity is a serious and life-threatening one. The effect in question might not occur in the animal species originally used in testing, or, in fact, in any animal species at all. Furthermore, the incidence in man may be so low that the toxicity did not have the chance to appear during the clinical trials, which normally involve no more than a few thousand patients.

For these reasons, surveillance must be continued for years after the release of a new drug to the medical profession. Reports of unexpected adverse reactions may come from practising physicians who can contact the drug firm involved and/or write (in the USA) to the Office of

Epidemiology and Biostatistics; or from hospital-based pharmacy and therapeutics committees who have special forms to be forwarded to the FDA. These essentially voluntary systems of reporting have not proved too successful. Few physicians seem motivated to report adverse effects with new drugs, and many (estimated at 40%) are even unaware that any such system exists. Other countries, e.g., UK, Canada, New Zealand, Denmark, Sweden, have legally mandated reporting systems, and these seem to work better.

A good example of a rare toxicity is the potentially fatal aplastic anaemia produced by the antibiotic chloramphenicol (Chloromycetin). This serious reaction occurs only about once in 30,000 courses of treatment with the drug, so it took two to three years of clinical use before it became obvious. Practolol (Eraldin), a so-called beta-blocker, was marketed in the UK in 1970 for the treatment of certain types of cardiovascular disease. It remained in wide use for four years before it was found to produce a curious group of symptoms known as the *oculomucocutaneous syndrome*. Skin, eyes, inner ear and peritoneal cavity were severely affected. Some patients went blind, and others required surgery and died as a consequence. The drug was immediately withdrawn from general medical use in 1974, and it is now reserved for emergency injection in special cases of disorder of the heart rhythm. Fortunately, there are other comparable agents in this particular group of drugs, and these can be administered without this risk.

The Research Director of ICI Pharmaceuticals (the firm which developed the drug) described this unforeseen side-effect as a "bolt from the blue", since the drug had been thoroughly tested on animals as well as clinically, and, moreover, had been approved by the UK Committee on Safety of Medicines. This case illustrates well many of the pitfalls faced by the drug industry in the promotion of new medicines. It seems that there is no animal species which would have revealed the undesirable syndrome during initial testing. Moreover, in man the syndrome is not only rare, but is thought to occur in a select minority of patients who show a special sensitivity to the drug based on immunological mechanisms.[3]

A more recent example of a drug that eventually had to be withdrawn (at least in the UK) is the benzodiazepine derivative triazolam (Halcion). This sleeping drug (hypnotic) was marketed by Upjohn Co. in 1983, and it is said that more than 43 million prescriptions of the drug have been written in the US. By 1991 triazolam had revealed some potentially dangerous side-effects of a psychiatric nature, e.g., loss of memory, and depression possibly leading to suicide, effects not observed with the many other benzodiazepines on the market. In this case, however, the outcome appears not to have been entirely a surprise to Upjohn, who admitted that in 1972 they had supplied the FDA with *incomplete* data in their application for approval.[4]

All these unfortunate examples might suggest that there are some good arguments for fewer animal tests and more and earlier clinical trials in man. However, as the American pharmacologist Bernard B. Brodie pointed out, all men (and women) are not equal in their response to drugs.[5] The human race shows some striking differences within the species in this respect, leading to clinically important consequences. Many of these variations are now thought to be related to genetically determined differences in rates and pathways of drug metabolism.

A classic case is the existence of two kinds of patients differing in the rate at which they inactivate in the body the drug isoniazid (used in treating tuberculosis). The inactivation occurs by adding an acetyl group to the drug molecule (acetylation). There are *slow inactivators* and *fast inactivators*, and the drug will clearly remain longer in the slow inactivators and so be more likely to produce adverse effects. However, the nature of the toxicities produced is not altered in any way. In populations of Western European origin, who first received isoniazid, slow inactivators make up about 55% of the total. Later, it turned out that other ethnic groups show a much lower percentage of slow inactivators, e.g., 15% in Japanese and only 5% in Eskimos.

The problem here arises from variations in the levels of the acetylating enzyme in the liver. Findings of this nature have, over the past 40 years, led to the development of the specialized branch of pharmacology known as pharmacogenetics, or the study of the influence of heredity on the response to clinically useful drugs. This term was first coined in 1962 by F. Vogel, and developed systematically by W. Kalow in his book *Pharmacogenetics* published in 1962.[6]

In some populations, certain enzyme deficiencies or abnormalities are present in a substantial proportion of individuals. One of the best known of these is a deficiency of an enzyme in the red blood cells called glucose-6-phosphate dehydrogenase (G6PD). Certain common drugs, normally relatively harmless, may cause haemolysis (the breakdown of red blood cells) in subjects with G6PD deficiency. It was discovered during World War II that, when American soldiers were given prophylactic doses of the antimalarial drug primaquine, some of them developed severe or even fatal haemolysis. The victims were derived ethnically from Mediterranean populations (e.g., Greeks, Sicilians, Sardinians), or African (e.g., Blacks, Puerto Ricans). Since that time, many other drugs have been reported to induce haemolysis in this deficiency, e.g., sulphonamides, phenacetin, chloramphenicol. The Africans tend to show a mild enzyme deficiency (8–20% of normal levels), while those of Mediterranean origin have a more severe deficiency (down to 0–4% of normal). Other variants of the condition are found in East and Southeast Asia, e.g., India, Thailand, Malaysia, Indonesia, Papua New Guinea and southern China.

Interestingly, in populations living round the Mediterranean, a tendency to develop haemolytic anaemia after eating broad beans has been well-known since classical times. The condition was termed favism from the botanical name of the bean *Vicea faba* (or *fava*). The Greek philosopher Pythagoras (flourished around 540–510 B.C.) forbade his followers to eat beans. The active principle in the bean is vicine which inhibits the activity of G6PD.

It is curious, and ironical, that it was an antimalarial drug which first revealed the syndrome. G6PD deficiency is thought to have developed by selection over the centuries as a protection against malaria. The malaria parasite does not flourish in the abnormal red cells, and consequently those carrying the enzyme defect were enabled to survive epidemics of the mosquito-borne disease. This, of course, explains its geographic distribution in areas where malaria was widespread in the past. The condition sickle cell anaemia also protects against malaria and is common in the same geographical areas, but is caused by an abnormal haemoglobin and not to G6PD deficiency. As a result, the red cells take on a deformed sickle-like shape.

Genetically determined G6PD deficiency is more common in males, and liable to be more severe, because the trait is sex-linked through the X-chromosome. This means that affected males have a single population of enzyme-deficient red cells, whereas most females (the so-called heterozygous ones) have two sorts of red cells, one normal and the other abnormal. Since only the abnormal cells are drug sensitive, drug-induced haemolysis in females is usually mild and unimportant clinically. When it comes to drug action, nature does not necessarily believe in the equality of the sexes.

Another pharmacogenetic trait, fortunately rare, can cause trouble during the administration of the drug succinylcholine (Scoline). This agent is a muscle relaxant valuable for brief surgical procedures, and is short-acting because it is rapidly destroyed in the blood by an enzyme known as plasma cholinesterase. Genetic abnormalities of this serum enzyme may cause a considerable slowing of the rate of inactivation of the drug. Since the muscles involved in breathing are affected by this muscle relaxant, and there is no immediate antidote to excess of it in the blood, respiratory difficulties and even asphyxia may develop and give concern to the anaesthetist in charge of the patient. The abnormality is clinically important in roughly one in 2,500 people of European origin, but uncommon in Africans and very rare in oriental populations.

Tests were devised by Kalow and Genest in 1957 for the detection of this abnormality in surgical patients so that the anaesthetist is aware of the situation. The atypical cholinesterase is less strongly inhibited by a local anaesthetic agent dibucaine (Nupercaine) than the normal enzyme (20% as compared with 80% for equal concentrations of dibucaine). The degree of inhibition provides the so-called dibucaine number, which quantitates the enzyme deficiency.[7]

These genetically based differences in reactions to drugs among various ethnic groups are still not as fully investigated as they should be. Most clinical trials are performed on Caucasian subjects, but after approval the drugs are sold, often aggressively, all over the world. Surprising toxicities may, therefore, turn up in non-Caucasians, and this is likely to happen more and more in the future as the spate of synthetic drugs continues to flood global markets.

It is only fair to add that reputable drug firms would be happy to sponsor more clinical trials among diverse racial groups, but modern facilities for studies of this kind are not always available in the regions concerned. Perhaps, also, a degree of ill-informed antagonism to such trials may exist on the grounds that they are thought to be a sort of neo-colonialist exploitation of the developing countries: "trying it out on the natives".

7

Unforeseen Dangers

The ingenuity of man has ever been fond of exerting
itself to varied forms and combinations of medicines.

William Withering (1785)

Certain extraneous and unforeseen factors can influence the human
response to a new drug, and these may also have to be kept in mind during
the early years of its therapeutic application. Some of these are: the route
of administration (whether oral or parenteral); the administration of one or
more other drugs at the same time (polypharmacy) leading to possible
adverse interactions; the condition of the recipient, e.g., malnutrition,
disease or age; and environmental factors such as exposure to chemicals in
food or to industrial toxins.

Many of these factors are related to alterations in the levels and
activities of the enzymes in the liver which modify (metabolize) drugs
chemically. Often the overall effect is merely to make necessary an
adjustment in dosage, and there is usually no change in the nature of the
side-effects produced. Those who live in traffic-polluted cities, smoke
cigarettes or both, inhale certain complex hydrocarbons known as
benzpyrene derivatives, and these substances can increase the levels of the
drug-metabolizing enzymes in the liver. These people, therefore, tend to
require somewhat larger doses of a drug because it will be more rapidly
metabolized in their livers.

Some chemicals ingested in food, e.g., insecticides which persisted
after spraying of crops, can also accelerate the metabolism of drugs
through liver enzyme induction. This effect with an insecticide like
chlorophenothane (DDT) can be long-lasting, because DDT is a very

fat-soluble substance which is taken up and stored in our adipose (fatty) tissues for many years. In other words, DDT has a very long half-life ($t_{1/2}$, see p. 87) estimated as between 200 and 1000 days or longer.[1] In the early 1980s , Britons and Americans had high levels of DDT in their body fats, though these have since declined. Apart from the effects on drug metabolism, which can be easily taken care of by increasing the dose of the therapeutic agent in question, these human levels of DDT do not seem to cause any harm. However, DDT is now widely banned, but mainly because of its effect on the ecological food chain which can eventually lead to impairment of the reproductive capacity of birds such as hawks and eagles (see Chap. 15, p. 105). It has been replaced with organophosphate insecticides having a brief $t_{1/2}$, but these also have their own toxicity.

Levels of drug-metabolizing enzymes may be depressed by factors such as malnutrition and outright starvation, and by some diseases of the liver. In these circumstances, a little more care is required since the usual dose of a drug in healthy patients may now amount to a relative overdosage, and there is a greater danger of coming into the toxic range. Newborn infants and elderly people may also metabolize drugs more slowly for the same reasons and with similar results. This effect is also enhanced in many such patients because of immature or impaired kidney function, slowing the excretion of the active metabolites.

Potentially far more serious problems arise from the unexpected interactions of a new drug with another drug or other drugs given at the same time. Polypharmacy, or multiple drug administration, is especially prevalent in hospital practice. A study in 1970 indicated that 40% of in-patients were receiving six or more drugs. However, some drug interactions are beneficial and deliberately exploited by the medical practitioner. A combination of drugs, for example, is often more effective in the treatment of tuberculosis, AIDS, hypertension or cancer than the single agents alone. An antidote may be a drug given intentionally to reverse the action of an overdose of another drug, e.g., naloxone counteracts the dangerous effects of too much morphine.

However, many of the special drug combinations marketed by the pharmaceutical industry have little therapeutic justification. Their cost is often exorbitant, and the doctor cannot vary the proportions of the individual components according to the needs and response of the patient. One possible argument in their favour is that the patient is at least spared the swallowing of many separate pills every day.

Drug interactions of a dangerous kind are more likely to occur when a patient needs multiple drug therapy for several disorders. So long as these drugs are being administered by one physician, he will, or should, be alert to this possibility and act accordingly. The trouble is that many patients may be self-administering over-the-counter (OTC) preparations and failing to inform their doctor; they may be consulting more than one doctor for their various ailments, and again not keeping all of them fully informed; or they may thoughtlessly accept and take left-over drugs from well-meaning friends or relatives. It is not commonly realized that some herbal preparations, e.g., St. John's Wort (*Hypericum perforatum*) often self-administered for mild depression, may interact with medicines prescribed by the doctor (and the patient may not think it important to inform him). The active principle or principles of the herb can stimulate the levels of drug-metabolizing enzymes in the liver, thereby decreasing the blood levels of drugs acted on by those enzymes, e.g., the blood-thinning agent warfarin (Coumadin), cyclosporin which prevents transplant rejection, the anti-asthma drug theophylline, certain drugs used to treat AIDS, and oral contraceptives. It may be necessary, therefore, to stop the St. John's Wort or increase the dose of the affected drug.[2]

The kind of remedies casually picked up at the supermarket, e.g., antacids, mild analgesics, nasal decongestants, are by themselves relatively harmless in reasonable dosage. Unfortunately, some of them may adversely interact with the more potent prescription drugs, and it is vitally important that the attending physician be told of any OTC drugs or preparations being taken, however trivial they might seem to the patient.

It should be remembered, too, that the ethyl alcohol in alcoholic drinks is a chemical with marked pharmacological actions, and therefore by strict definition a drug. A not uncommon interaction which can be unpleasant, and even fatal, occurs when people drink alcohol excessively and then take sedatives, hypnotics or tranquillisers. All these drugs individually depress the nervous system, and taken together there is an additive or synergistic effect which can lead to coma, cessation of breathing and death.

In synergism there may be simple summation of the effects of the several drugs taken, or one drug may actually potentiate the actions of the others. Synergism can take place between anticoagulant drugs and the OTC drug aspirin. The anticoagulant drugs are given intentionally to make the circulating blood less likely to clot and so help to prevent thrombosis in the blood vessels. What is seldom realized by many patients is that aspirin has a similar pharmacological activity, and if the patient is taking it regularly the combined anticoagulant effect could lead to a fatal haemorrhage.

More complex than simple synergism are the interactions based on enzyme inhibition. A famous example of this is the interaction between drugs known as monoamine oxidase inhibitors and certain substances present in OTC preparations for relieving the symptoms of a cold. The monoamine oxidase inhibitors became popular some years ago among psychiatrists for the treatment of certain types of severe mental depression. These drugs inhibit the activity of the important enzyme monoamine oxidase, which inactivates adrenaline and other active amines in the body. The enzyme also inactivates the amines, present in, and absorbed from, a number of nasal decongestant sprays which act by constricting the blood vessels in the nasal mucosa, (e.g., phenylephrine, xylometazoline). If the enzyme is blocked, the absorbed amines are not destroyed in the tissues and may cause a marked and even catastrophic general rise in the blood pressure. The recreational drugs cocaine and Ecstasy may have similar effects in those taking monoamine oxidase inhibitors.

Similar amines with an effect on blood pressure, e.g., tyramine, are present in quite large amounts in some foods. In the early days of the monoamine oxidase inhibitors, certain patients developed mysterious episodes or crises of hypertension with headache, photophobia, neck stiffness and collapse, even though no other drugs were being taken. An observant pharmacist whose wife was on the monoamine oxidase inhibitor tranylcypromine noticed that the crises seemed to follow her favourite cheese supper. Another patient on this drug died in 1965 after eating a cheese soufflé. Eventually the interaction was attributed, with some incredulity on the part of the physicians, to the tyramine in the cheese.

In a drug-free normal person, the tyramine in the cheese would be inactivated before it had the chance to raise the blood pressure. Apart from cheeses, especially those of the *aged* kind like Brie, foods like beer, wines, chicken livers, pickled herrings, snails, yeast extracts (e.g., Marmite), canned figs, broad beans and chocolate also contain large quantities of tyramine or similar amines such as dihydroxyphenylalanine (dopa), and can interact with the monoamine oxidase inhibitors. Aged cheeses and yeast products are the most dangerous as they may contain 10 mg or more tyramine per serving.

We may now return to the vexed question, raised in Chap. 4, p. 39, of who should bear the responsibility, and pay compensation, for these various unexpected adverse effects of drugs. Clearly, if the toxicity of a new drug can be definitely blamed on the negligence of the manufacturer during production and testing, then the firm involved must accept complete responsibility and should compensate the victims. Equally, if a physician wrongly prescribes a drug with known serious toxicity for a trivial or irrelevant condition, then he must bear the liability.

But it is the unique factors inseparable from the use of drugs in medical practice which pose the really tricky social and legal problems. First, drug treatment is almost always potentially hazardous due to the essential nature of drugs as *selective poisons.*

Second, the degree of hazard acceptable in a drug is related to the severity of the disease to be treated. Highly toxic agents can be given for the treatment of cancer or AIDS because the risk of withholding treatment is likely to be even more serious.

Third, the establishment of a cause-effect relationship in drug toxicity is often very difficult, and may be impossible.

All these have led to a growing opinion in civilized communities that there should be some kind of automatic compensation for every type of personal injury, including those caused by drugs, i.e., a *no-fault liability* scheme not dependent on absolute proof of blame.

D.R. Laurence, formerly Professor of Pharmacology and Therapeutics at University College, London, has outlined a possible solution to this knotty problem.[3] If new drugs undergoing clinical testing cause any adverse effects during Phase II (limited trials) or serious toxicities during Phase III (extended trials), then the sponsor (usually the manufacturer) should be prepared to accept full liability.

Unexpected toxicities that turn up later from drugs already tested and approved for medical use cannot in all fairness be blamed on the manufacturer. In the case of practolol (see p. 49) ICI acknowledged moral, but not legal, liability for the bizarre toxicity, and paid compensation to the approximately one thousand patients who claimed to be affected. Many would regard this as justified in view of the strong promotional pressures exerted on the medical profession by the pharmaceutical industry.

However, Laurence suggests that this kind of situation would be better dealt with by a no-fault liability scheme, operated by government through quick-acting tribunals. These tribunals would merely have to be satisfied that the drug was beyond reasonable doubt the cause of the injury; that the injury was serious; and that the type of injury was not sufficiently common with that drug to have deterred the doctor from administering it to the patient. The tribunal would determine a fair compensation to the victim, and expect at least partial reimbursement from the manufacturer, supplier and prescriber, as appropriate.

This is, perhaps, far from the perfect answer. It seems irrational, for example, that someone should be compensated for an accident due to drug treatment, and yet not be compensated for the accident of the disease itself. There are obviously enormous difficulties in finding a logical solution to the immensely complex moral and legal problems raised by drug toxicity in modern society.

8

What's in a Name?

The objective of society ought properly to be toward
fewer and fewer drugs rather than more and more,
and fewer doctors also, for that matter,
until eventually it can get along with none.

[Attributed] to René Dubos

Here is a simple quiz. What do the following drugs, all available in the USA or Canada, have in common: Deltasone, Meticorten, Orasone, Sterapred, Winpred and Prednicen-M?

The answer is rather disturbing; they are all preparations of exactly the same drug, prednisone. This is a useful and potent synthetic adreno-corticoid, i.e., a drug which imitates more or less the actions of the steroid hydrocortisone normally produced in the adrenal cortex. However, chronic administration of high doses of prednisone can cause a number of serious side-effects ranging from hypertension through osteoporosis and collapsed vertebrae to "moon face".

Preparations of the popular analgesic (pain-killing) drug aceta-minophen or paracetamol are listed in *The Complete Drug Reference* (published by the American Consumers Union, 1991 Edition, with the authority of the US Pharmacopeial Convention, Inc.) under 84 different names in the US and 21 in Canada.[1] Clearly, a new drug must be given a name for identification and communication, but why such a confusion of many names?

Since any drug is a chemical compound, it possesses a full chemical name, but unfortunately this rarely trips easily off the tongue. Even the most seasoned organic chemist prefers to use a convenient abbreviation, known as the trivial name. For example, the full chemical name for adrenaline is dihydroxyphenylmethylaminoethanol.

The drug firm originally marketing the chemical as a drug will select a proprietary or trade name, and later on, when other firms come to manufacture the same drug, they, naturally, will wish to coin their own special proprietary name. Meanwhile, various official bodies meet to decide on a non-proprietary, official or approved name for use in formularies and pharmacopoeias, and in the teaching of pharmacology and therapeutics to medical students, pharmacists, etc. This is sometimes, but inaccurately, described as the generic name, a term which should strictly refer only to a category of drugs such as suphonamides or barbiturates.

A drug occasionally used for the treatment of high blood pressure has the full chemical name of levo-alpha-methyldihydroxyphenylalanine, and the more manageable trivial name of L-alphamethyldopa. In this case, the approved name is a further abbreviation of the chemical name: methyldopa. Trade names listed in *The Complete Drug Reference* are Aldomet, Apo-Methyldopa, Dopamet and Novomedopa.

In this book, by the way, approved names will be spelled with a small initial letter, e.g., prednisone; and trade names with a capital, e.g., Deltasone.

The chemical name is predetermined by the molecular structure of the compound, and the approved name is often a shortened, though not necessarily more euphonious, version of this. Trade or proprietary names, on the other hand, are selected by the drug firms to trip lightly off the tongues of doctors of all races and nationalities, even those unused to polysyllabic words or the clash of harsh, unfamiliar consonants.

The number of modern drugs and preparations existing worldwide is difficult to estimate, but may exceed 50,000, and is growing annually. The search for proprietary names by the pharmaceutical firms has, therefore, become quite a problem. In an article which appeared in the *New Yorker* in 1956, a drug firm spokesman was reported as saying, "thinking up names has been driving us cuckoo around here ... A good trade name carries a lot of weight with doctors ... they're more apt to write a prescription for a drug whose name is short and easy to spell and pronounce, but has an impressive medical ring." This firm had used a computer to produce a dictionary of 42,000 nonsense words of an appropriate scientific look and sound. The spokesman commented, "We don't know what proportion of names is unpronounceable ... how many are obscene, either in English or in other languages ... The names which look and sound medically seductive will go into a stockpile and await the inexorable proliferation of new drugs."

The burden of many drug names is one that weighs heavily on the medical student's memory, and continues to confuse the practitioner throughout his whole clinical career. Moreover, the drugs he learned about as a student may well have become obsolete and replaced by new, but not necessarily improved, products with new official names and an equal multiplicity of trade names. The alphabetical index of the *Physicians' Desk Reference*[2] contains nearly 6,954 names of drugs and preparations in its 1999 edition, most of them trade names. Not surprisingly, many of these, even the approved names, look or sound quite similar to the practiced medical anglophone. It is amazing that the following kinds of disasters do not occur more frequently.

A theatre sister in the UK asked for one gram of procaine from the hospital dispensary, and was given Percaine in error.[3] (Both drugs are local anesthetics, but Percaine is much more potent weight for weight.) The patient who received an injection of the wrong drug went into convulsions and died fifteen minutes later. The dispenser was so sure that procaine and Percaine were one and the same drug that she did not bother to check. After this catastrophe, which took place in the late 1930s, the firm manufacturing Percaine changed the proprietary name in the UK to Nupercaine. The two drugs Losec and Lasix may not sound too alike, but bad writing by a hospital doctor in Belgium is said to have led to death of a patient. Losec (omeprazole) is a drug which diminishes the secretion of acid in the stomach, and Lasix is a diuretic (increasing urine flow) and an antihypertensive drug. The patient was on Losec and was prescribed a further dose, but misreading led to the fatal administration of Lasix instead. In the USA, the FDA eventually mandated that Losec be renamed Prilosec, hardly a very radical change. In 1991, omeprazole was still called Losec in Canada.

Only, it would seem, extraordinarily bad handwriting could lead to confusion between amiodarone (for congestive heart failure) and amrinone (for heart rhythm disturbances); Covera HS (for high blood pressure) and Provera (a synthetic variant of the female hormone progesterone); and Norvasc (amlodipine, an antihypertensive drug) and Navane (thiothixine, a drug used in some mental conditions).

On the other hand, gross dissimilarity in trade names can lull doctors into thinking they refer to completely different drugs. There is the possibly apochryphal story of the German practitioner who treated a patient with the new drug Paraxin, a free sample presented to him by a persuasive representative from firm A. When the patient returned two weeks later, no better, the doctor switched to Leukomycin, a gift from firm B. This misguided doctor was blissfully unaware that Paraxin and Leukomycin were both trade names for the antibiotic chloramphenicol.

Such problems apart, it is not surprising, therefore, that pharmacologists prefer to use approved names in their teaching, and attempt to encourage in future doctors a life-long habit of avoiding proprietary names. Unfortunately, this is apt to be a losing battle, since even the hospital consultants, who train the students in their clinical years, readily fall into the trap of employing the trade names of their favourite drugs, and practitioners in the outside world are too much under the influences of the drug firm representatives (detail men) to use the approved names.

Approved names are determined by WHO and almost always universally accepted, but there is one unfortunate exception that is fully discussed by Jeffrey K. Aronson in a recent issue of the *British Medical Journal*.[4] The adrenergic transmitter adrenaline (see Chap. 19, p. 133) has been known in the USA since 1897 as epinephrine. (Linguistically they mean the same; adrenaline is derived from Latin and epinephrine from Greek.) Most of the rest of the world, except Canada, Spain and Japan, prefer to use the designation adrenaline, but the WHO's recommended non-proprietary name (rINN) is epinephrine. In 1992, a European Union Commission issued a directive to conform to the WHO'S rINN. This directive was intended to be fully implemented by the UK Medicines Control Agency by 1998, but in September 2000 it was still not in force. Aronson explains that using the name epinephrine could lead to some unfortunate mix-ups, e.g., between the stimulant drug ephedrine and epinephrine.

But the approved name has many advantages. Though possibly tongue-twisting, it often gives the doctor some clue to the class of drug he is proposing to prescribe. Drugs sold under official names are sometimes far less expensive than similar preparations sold under proprietary names. Soluble aspirin USP is cheaper than the many fancy preparations claimed, usually on precious little evidence, to "act faster", "have built-in stomach protection", "help the hurt stop hurting" and other vague blandishments.

Another important point is that if a doctor prescribes a drug under the approved name, the pharmacist has the option of supplying the patient with any particular brand of that drug which he has in stock. If the doctor prescribes a proprietary name with the proviso "do not substitute", then the pharmacist is obliged to supply that brand, and if it is not immediately available he will have to waste time obtaining it.

To advocate the use of approved names is frowned upon by the drug firms, who have, of course, a strong brand loyalty. However, all reputable firms today are scrupulous about quality control of their products, especially in matters relating to purity and accuracy of dosage. (This may not be a safe assumption in some third world countries, and certainly was not so in the past.)

The pressures from drug firms to persuade doctors to prescribe specifically their own brand names are understandable, and, not so many years ago, the realization of the importance of a factor known as biological availability presented them with a heaven-sent scientific argument for this. Naturally they were not slow to take advantage of it.

If a drug is injected directly into the veins of a patient so that all of it arrives at the tissues where it acts pharmacologically, then the biological availability (bioavailability, for short) is said to be 100%. If a drug is swallowed, or injected by other routes, some of it may be lost or destroyed before it reaches the circulation, and in that case its bioavailability would be something less than 100%. Different drugs might be expected to have different bioavailabilities, but the *same* drug would, one would think, show the same bioavailability, i.e., a constant proportion should reach the tissues on which it acts, assuming that one uses exactly the same route of administration. Some disturbing experiences with the drug digoxin showed that this was not, in fact, the case. Four different digoxin preparations, given by mouth, produced as much as a sevenfold variation in the levels of the drug in the bloodstream.

It turned out that certain factors in the manufacture of the digoxin tablets, e.g., the particle size of the active drug, the nature of the inert substance or excipient which makes up the bulk of the tablet and the hardness of the tablet itself were responsible for the significant variations in the observed bioavailability. In practical terms, this means that if a patient is stabilized on a certain dose of digoxin from Firm A, and then the physician changes to digoxin from Firm B, an increase of bioavailability would lead to unexpected toxicity; and conversely, a decrease of bioavailability would lead to inadequate therapeutic effect. This provides an argument for sticking to one particular preparation, and ensuring this by prescribing the trade name.

The argument was a trifle blunted when it was discovered that different batches of digoxin made by the same firm could also differ alarmingly in bioavailability. Today, most reputable firms would, and should, feel under an obligation to standardize very carefully the pharmaceutical bioavailability of their preparations. Nevertheless, it might be prudent, with repeat prescriptions, to ensure the same brand each time by using a trade name, especially for patients on long-term therapy, with a precisely adjusted dose of a potentially toxic agent.

In the next chapter, something must be said about how the drug industry promotes the sales of its cornucopia of seductively named products to the public and to the medical profession.

9

A Profit Without Honour

The drug companies are doing what they can to make as much money as they can.
This is the behaviour you would have expected.

Sidney Wolfe,
Director of the Health Research Group,
a consumer advocacy organization
in Washington DC (1991).

In 1961, a scandal blew up in Britain over drug prices. The Minister of Health in the Conservative government, Mr. Enoch Powell, in an attempt to curb the spiralling costs of the National Health Service, awarded a big contract to a new drug firm (DDSA Pharmaceuticals) for supplies of the antibiotic agent tetracycline.

This enterprising firm did not itself manufacture tetracycline, but imported it from Italy or from countries in Eastern Europe, where patents on drugs were not permitted, or not recognized. All DDSA Pharmaceuticals had to do was to weigh out the required dosage, make it into tablets or capsules, and package the product. In spite of having to pay an import duty, and allowing themselves a reasonable profit, they were able to sell to the government for almost one-tenth the price charged by the patent holders, the original discoverers of tetracycline. The implication was that the patentees' rights allowed them to monopolize the market in tetracycline, and so they were able to maintain the price at an artificially high level.

It will be remembered that, at roughly the same time as this particular cat was being let out of the bag, the thalidomide disaster was about to explode on an unsuspecting public. Also, in the USA, a Senate Sub-committee on Anti-Trust and Monopoly, which had been deliberating for some years, had just brought out its searching report (known as the Kefauver Report) on the inner workings of the pharmaceutical industry. All these events led to considerable public unease over the manufacture and testing of drugs, and their application to medical practice. In 1965, the well-known journalist and television personality Brian Inglis published an outspoken survey of the pharmaceutical industry called *Drugs, Doctors and Disease.*[1]

Inglis tells the tetracycline story, and also describes how the first hint of price-fixing in the US came to light in 1951 when the husband of one of the Federal Trade Commission's staff developed a sore throat, and his doctor prescribed chloramphenicol. (*Note*: a potentially very toxic drug like chloramphenicol should *never* be given for such a trivial condition. However, the dangers of chloramphenicol were only begun to be realized around 1953.) The patient stopped at a drug store to fill his prescription, and found that chloramphenicol tablets were 50¢ each. Thinking this excessive, he telephoned his doctor and asked if a cheaper antibiotic was available. The doctor suggested two alternatives, Aureomycin or Terramycin. These also turned out to be exactly 50¢ a tablet, a remarkable coincidence in view of the fact that the three drugs were made by three different firms. This suggestive evidence of high prices, and of price-fixing between firms, was reported to the Federal Trade Commission (FTC), but little was done about it until 1957 when Senator Estes Kefauver took over as Chairman of the Senate Sub-committee on Anti-Trust and Monopoly.

Brian Inglis describes in detail the proceedings of the Kefauver Committee, and the startling revelations of price-fixing and excessive profit-taking among the leading American drug firms. These findings also caused much concern in the UK because of the take-over of many British firms by American ones, and the creation of powerful multinational organizations. The international character of many drug companies naturally bedevils control by individual governments, and is, perhaps, regarded by those companies as one defence against the threat of nationalization by possible Labour or Socialist administrations outside the USA.

The Kefauver Committee also looked closely into the promotional activities of the pharmaceutical industry, and these are of greater interest to us here.

Dr. A. Console, basing his evidence to the Committee on his previous experience as a medical director of Squibb, divided the products of the industry into four groups: effective drugs prescribed only for patients who need them; drugs prescribed for patients who do not need them; drugs from which patients derive no benefit; and drugs which have a greater potential for harm than for good. The extraordinary thing was, said Dr. Console, that less money was spent on the development and promotion of the first group than of the other three. It was this, no doubt, which led Milton Silverman, Philip R. Lee and Mia Lydecker to make the following acid comment in their book *Prescriptions for Death* (1982): "If a man should make a better mousetrap ... the world will beat a path to his door. But if the new mousetrap is not better than the old, what then? Facing this kind of dilemma, the drug industry has found a remarkably satisfactory answer: double the advertising budget."[2]

The fact is that much of the money for so-called research, which the drug firms claim as an excuse for the high cost of drugs, is used to improve packaging and to promote marketing and publicity. It is not devoted to seeking the epoch-making breakthrough in treatment. This is a rare event, anyway, and many new products put on the market are simply minor variants of an approved drug; or established drugs with unnecessary or even undesirable additives; or combinations of approved drugs for special therapeutic purposes.

It is possible, for instance, to circumvent patent rights by synthesizing a drug the molecule of which is structurally only slightly different from one already manufactured by a rival firm. The highly qualified chemists employed by the drug companies are adept at this game of molecular roulette, and the variants produced are sometimes referred to as "me-too" drugs. Every firm, for example, must have its own lucrative antihistamine agent, however little it differs in action (and side effects) from others on the market.

This is not to say that minor structural changes in a drug molecule can never lead to striking improvements, with increased efficacy and reduced toxicity, but such an outcome of the gamble of molecular roulette is uncommon.

Additives to widely-used drugs like the antibiotics are claimed, often on flimsy evidence, to improve absorption into the circulation, or in some other subtle way to increase the efficacy of the active agent. Even if the additive did really help to produce higher blood levels with the same dose of the active drug, it would surely be easier (and probably cheaper) to give a slightly larger dose of the unadulterated agent. Combinations of active drugs can be hazardous, as they may, by providing thoughtless shot-gun therapy, encourage doctors to evade the discipline of making a firm diagnosis, and (in the case of antibiotics) to risk the development of resistant strains of bacteria.

Since few of these special preparations represent a serious advance in therapeutics, and this would soon be realized by the medical profession, the aim of the drug companies is the quick kill with the quick pill, employing high-pressure salesmanship to garner short-term profits.

Most of the promotional activities of the drug firms are, of course, aimed at the medical profession: direct mailing of informational literature, advertisements in medical journals and paramedical publications, videotapes, free samples of drugs, and even free gifts such as golf balls with the firm logo or $15,000-worth of computer equipment. This bombardment is followed up by the personal visit of the detail man (USA) or drug rep (UK), who is trained to coat his silver-tongued panegyric of the merchandise with a plausible pharmacological veneer.[3]

A witness told the Kefauver Committee that, if the daily load of drug circulars and samples mailed to physicians in the USA was addressed to one city, it would require two railroad mailvans, 110 large mail trucks and 800 mailmen to effect delivery. Afterwards, over 25 garbage trucks would be needed to haul it away to the city dump for burning, and the blaze would be visible on a clear day for 50 miles. All this promotion, which costs the industry more than $5 billion a year in the US alone, is for the so-called ethical products, the prescription drugs that are advertised only to the medical profession. The advertising of over-the-counter drugs in the various media is, of course, on a much less sophisticated level, and designed for lay consumption.

The drug firms also have more subtle, and sometimes apparently more high-minded, gimmicks for promoting their products, e.g., financing drug trials among general practitioners, or organizing a conference in suitably idyllic surroundings with lavish recreational facilities laid on. One firm was reported to have rented 3,000 acres of marshland in order to entertain 700 doctors to a weekend of duck shooting. Abbott Laboratories in the early 1980s boosted their new tranquillizer Tranxene by inviting doctors to a night at the opera in New York, at which singers performed scenes portraying neurotic episodes from well-known operas. After the performances, the psychological conditions were described in detail and the new drug was recommended as the medication of choice.

Basic research publications in reputable scientific and medical journals are not always what they seem. The Kefauver Committee discovered that some papers submitted under the name of a respected medical investigator were in fact prepared by the staff of a pharmaceutical company, and contained subtle propaganda for their new drug. Such papers are then utilized as supposedly independent references for the firm's drug advertizing literature.

Although the revelations of the Kefauver Committee have had some long-term effects on the behaviour of the drug industry, a 1990 Senate Labor and Human Resources Committee chaired by Sen. Edward M. Kennedy made it clear that many of the same problems remain today. This committee considered three important questions: (1) Where does good, aggressive marketing of potentially life-saving products cross the line into bribery? (2) Are the costs of free gifts to doctors being passed on to patients? (3) Who, if not the companies that developed them, should be educating doctors about new medicines? In connection with question 3, a Seattle internist recently claimed that the "pharmaceutical companies now subsidize virtually all continuing education for doctors." There would seem here to be a serious conflict of interests.

Another widespread, but surely unethical, gambit is to *get at* the doctors indirectly through the drug-swallowing public. This can involve the planting in the nation's press of what appear to be news items informing the public of the development of a new drug, and giving details of its principal uses in medicine. These lead the patient to bring the existence of the new drug to the attention of the physician before very much is known about it, and to pressure him to use it instead of better-established therapy. As a result of these activities, the physician is urged to abandon the treatment he knows well, and use one which he has little or no experience with.

In November 1963, the London *Sunday Times* had an article headlined: "New British Drug is more Effective than Penicillin." At that time the results of clinical trials with this drug, cephalothin, had not even been released to the medical profession; and yet it contained phrases like "the perfect antibiotic"; "effective against a much wider range of germs than ordinary penicillin"; "remarkably free from poisonous effects in human beings". Another headline in a Hong Kong newspaper in 1981 read: "Super Drug put to Test". The short news item used expressions like: "a new group of superantibiotics", and contained the obligatory misprint (monobactams for monolactams), but it was clear from the final paragraph that clinical testing in human volunteers (Phase I) had only just begun.

Whether such press releases are deliberate promotional leaks on the part of the drug industry, or merely the scoops of an overly enthusiastic journalist not too familiar with the pitfalls of new drug therapy, is not always clear. But whichever they are, they have the undesirable effect of inciting the layman to attempt a half-baked dictation of drug treatment to his overworked and long-suffering doctor. The then Director of the FDA, Dr. David Kessler, introduced new regulations in 1991 to make it more difficult to get such promotional misinformation into print or on the air.

Since the scandals and revelations of the early 1960s and of more recent times, much serious thought has been given to the problems raised by the pressures exerted on the medical profession by the pharmaceutical industry on the one hand, and by the lay public on the other. Some of the possible answers to these dilemmas will be discussed in the next chapter.

10

Doctors' Dilemmas

[D]octors, if they will permit me to say so, are
ignorant — they are governed by names: so detached
they are from the process of making up drugs, which
used to be the special business of the ... profession.

Pliny, the Elder (23–79 AD), *Natural History*, 34.25

Pliny's comments were echoed, perhaps a trifle hypocritically, by a drug
firm President some 1900 years later. "It frightens me that the general
medical community throughout the world is largely influenced by slogans,
and its convictions are based on slogans." (quoted by Brian Inglis in *The
Diseases of Civilisation*, 1981).[1] This addiction to names and slogans,
which creates pressures on doctors to prescribe unnecessary, or untried and
possibly dangerous, drugs, is encouraged by the aggressive promotional
activities of the pharmaceutical industry, either directly or through their
patients.

We must now consider how the threat of legal and professional
restraint, and the availability of more accurate and reliable information,
have been applied in recent years to diminish the dangers and abuses
arising directly and indirectly from the profit-seeking propensities of the
powerful multinational drug companies.

In the 40 odd years that have elapsed since the thalidomide tragedy,
there is no doubt that the screening of new drugs for toxicity through
carefully controlled animal and human testing has been greatly improved.
Moreover, the pharmaceutical industry is now very much on the defensive
and is aware that its reputation as a source of wonder drugs is somewhat
tarnished. It bends over backwards to avoid the bad publicity that would

overwhelm it, especially in the developed countries, if a new drug were linked with serious adverse reactions. In addition, governmental and professional bodies have been set up to monitor reported toxicities for many years after a new drug is released, e.g., the FDA in the US and the UK Committee on Safety of Medicines (now incorporated into a European Union organization based in London). The World Health Organization (WHO) has also organized a research centre for international drug monitoring which collaborates with national centres in many countries.

Of course, this greatly increased concern for the careful monitoring of drug safety by government agencies and their committees, as well as by the drug companies themselves, has added enormously (some would say prohibitively) to the cost of developing new drugs. The pharmaceutical firms can hardly be blamed for passing on part of this to the patient, though there are some curious anomalies here, e.g., the US public is often charged more for the same drug than consumers in Canada or Europe.

Since the publication of the Kefauver Report, the more blatantly profiteering aspects of drug salesmanship have been, one hopes, checked in many countries by increasingly stringent government control. For example, in the US, a "maximum allowable cost" (MAC) programme was started in 1976 to fix the maximum price the government will pay for certain drugs supplied in connection with Medicare and Medicaid schemes. Promotional activities are also under supervision. The FDA has authority over ethical drug advertising, and the drug firms must submit their promotional material for review. The Federal Trade Commission (FTC) watches over-the-counter drug advertising on TV and in newspapers and magazines, and, as mentioned in Chap. 9 (p. 70), the FDA Director Dr. David Kessler introduced rigorous regulations for these agents in 1992. But we must remember that loopholes can always be found in the most carefully devised of laws and guidelines. An example of this recently surfaced. A drug approved as efficacious in one disease may have secondary applications which the drug firm can promote without any evidence that it is effective or safe for other conditions. The secondary use is known as *off-label* use. For example, the drug Retin-A is approved for treatment of acne, but not for the *off-label* removal of wrinkles in aging skin, a dubious cosmetic procedure. No doubt highly-paid company lawyers are busy seeking other ways around existing regulations.

So, can the Kefauver Report now be regarded as of historical interest only? Unfortunately, the profit-hunting leopard does not readily change his spots, even though, with governments breathing down his neck, he may find it expedient on occasions to resort to their cosmetic disguise. In those countries without strict legislation, and where medical personnel and facilities are grossly inadequate, the beast may still stalk his profits with spots unveiled. Some multinational drug companies continue to exaggerate claims of efficacy for their products, cover up potential hazards, and otherwise behave in a socially irresponsible fashion.[2]

Brian Inglis has reported hints of this kind of attitude revealed during a Kefauver hearing on a synthetic corticosteroid dexamethasone (Decadron).[3] Sen. Kefauver had asked the director of medical research of the firm involved whether the promotional claims of complete freedom from side effects were accurate. The director admitted they were not. Kefauver then asked the president of the company if, in this case, they should have made such boasts as: "Patient need is the main consideration – NO STEROID SIDE EFFECTS". The president quickly replied, "this particular ad is used by our international division"; and then no doubt bit his tongue as Kefauver snapped back, "you mean you make different claims abroad?" The director of medical research stepped in hurriedly to say, "we don't condone false statements either abroad or domestically." "All right", pursued the Senator, "would the Director accept the truth of a recent claim that no worrisome side effects attributable to Decadron had occurred as yet." We can imagine the hush as the director replied, "as of today, I would say it is not true."

For many years the United Nations has attempted to deal with these double standards in drug advertising and salesmanship. A journalist in 1972 observed that the UN, through its various agencies, was fighting an *undeclared war* on the multinational drug companies, and combating what the then Director General of the World Health Organization (WHO), Dr. Halfdan Mahler, called "*drug colonialism*". Dr. Mahler did not think that the battle would be easily won. He feared that any attempt to move towards a rational drug policy, especially in the undeveloped countries, would be opposed by the local medical establishment and the international drug industry.

The UN followed several strategies to improve the developing countries' self-reliance in drugs. The first was a WHO plan to devise a short-list of essential drugs for a particular country, thereby reducing the imports of non-essential and costly drugs. Needless to say, this scheme aroused considerable opposition from the pharmaceutical industry, but nevertheless has survived largely due to the support of an international coalition of consumer activists known as Health Action International

(HAI). A second scheme to cut prices by bulk buying of drugs was organized by the United Nations Conference on Trade and Development (UNCTAD). The United Nations Industrial Development Organization (UNIDO) encouraged local drug industry and the use to some degree of effective herbal medicines indigenous to the country concerned.

An article in the *World Health Forum* (WHO, Geneva, 1980) by Dr. V. T. Herat Gunaratne, Director of the WHO Regional Office for Southeast Asia in New Delhi, reported the successful efforts of Sri Lanka to reduce the costs of its imported drugs. He described the situation in the Third World countries in forceful terms: "The huge multinational drug companies … have been marketing their products for the last few decades in the developing countries, unmindful of the health needs and health priorities of these countries." In Tanzania, he wrote, "pharmaceutical salesmen are in a ratio of one to every four doctors." In Dar-es-Salaam, the amount spent by the commercial companies in the promotion of drugs exceeds the total budget for the Faculty of Medicine! These facts partly explain why, in developing countries, the drug budget as a percentage of total health expenditure tends to be high, ranging from 63.8% in Bangladesh to 18.8% in India. But in Sri Lanka by 1980 the figure had been reduced to a gratifyingly low 7.5%. How?

In the late fifties, the Sri Lanka government produced a Ceylon Hospital Formulary to guide the country's practitioners in their choice of drugs. The short-list of essential drugs was selected from those which could be obtained most cheaply (e.g., the tranquillizer diazepam was bought from an international source charging only one-fiftieth what was previously paid), and which would serve real social needs. A point made by Dr. Gunaratne was that, although "the giant multinationals are spending large sums of money on drug research, … their priorities are totally out of tune with the disease patterns in the developing countries. Whereas our problems are still largely the infectious diseases, research in Western countries is concentrated mainly on cancer chemotherapy, diseases of affluence and geriatrics."

It is certainly true that, although more than US$2 billion is said to be spent annually on drug research worldwide, only a very small proportion of these funds is directed to the discovery of improved drugs for treating important tropical diseases. As an editorial in the *British Medical Journal* said some years ago, the reasons for this state of affairs are simple: unless the market for the drug is likely to be large and the profits considerable, the pharmaceutical industry will just not bother to provide it.

The idea of saving money by using fewer, well-tried drugs has also been suggested for the UK where the cost of pharmaceutical services has represented about 10% of the national health expenditure for many years. Most doctors write about 75% of their prescriptions from about 100 preparations, even though the maximum number of preparations used by an individual doctor can be as high as 500. Obviously, the average practitioner does not require anything like the approximately 50,000 drugs and preparations now available, and the fewer he uses the more likely he is to be really familiar with all their actions and side effects.

The misdeeds of the multinationals, referred to above, should not blind us to the shortcomings of the domestic or national drug companies, many of which may aggressively promote drugs (e.g., enterovioform) that have been withdrawn by the bigger firms. Pharmaceutical products made and sold in some Third World countries often lack good quality control during production and distribution, and may even be counterfeit or fraudulent. This can be a serious problem.[4]

In spite of all that we have said above, it would be unfair to cast the drug industry as the only villain. A recent review in the *Lancet* of a book by Andrew Chetley, who was long a leading figure in and spokesman for HAI, pointed out that "there is no shortage of doctors to play Faust to [the Industry's] Mephistopheles." They are still only too willing to accept the bribes offered to them. On the other side, Chetley, in his book *A Healthy Business? World Health and the Pharmaceutical Industry*, detects recent industry efforts to improve adverse drug reaction monitoring, and to consult with consumer activist groups.[5]

The fact remains that the immediate and long-term protection of the public against the inescapable dangers of drugs lies firmly in the hands of the primary care physician, and depends ultimately on the quality of his educational background in pharmacology and therapeutics. If the training of doctors in those subjects is inadequate (as Brian Inglis said it was in 1965), then it is not surprising that the drug companies rush in to fill the vacuum, and take upon themselves the task of *educating* (or more tactfully, informing) the profession about drugs. Looked at from this point of view, it could surely be said that the medical profession gets the pharmaceutical industry it deserves.

Improvement in the education of doctors has always been, of course, a matter for the medical profession itself, since by long tradition all professions have the privilege of regulating their own affairs internally without governmental or other outside interference. Hence G.B. Shaw's remark, in the preface to his play *The Doctor's Dilemma*, that "every profession is a conspiracy against the laity". And as Thomas Szasz, the American psychiatrist turned iconoclast and anti-establishment gadfly, writes, "the professions thrive on jargon, mumbo-jumbo and keeping the public in the dark."

Fortunately, since 1965 there has been a gradual, if reluctant, acceptance by the medical establishment of the increasing importance of a thorough training in the principles of pharmacology and therapeutics for the undergraduate medical student. The new discipline of clinical pharmacology has become respectable (see Chap. 2, p. 23). It is also realized that education in the use of modern drugs must be continued throughout a doctor's career by means of refresher and other postgraduate courses. Moreover, professional organizations have attempted to keep the practising physician up-to-date and well-informed about drugs through the medium of publications such as the *British National Formulary, The Medical Letter* (USA) and the *Drug and Therapeutics Bulletin* (UK). These are, of course, quite independent of the pharmaceutical industry, and do not mince their words if they consider some new drugs to be unduly toxic, or no better than existing agents. Better trained and better informed doctors would not only be more effectively immunized against the promotional blandishments of the industry, but would also be more resistant to attempts at therapeutic dictation from their patients.

In the complex interrelationships between industry, profession and patients, there is also a need for better education of the general public. Thomas Szasz believes that even children of 12–13 could, and should, be taught in school the basic principles and facts of physiology, and of the major diseases and their treatment. His idea is to ensure in the doctor's office a rational and knowledgeable clientele who no longer demands the traditional role of the physician as priest-magician.

11

Journey to the Interior

> Doctors pour drugs of which they know little ...
> into human beings of whom they know nothing.
>
> Voltaire (1694–1778)

Over 200 years ago, at a time when medicaments were few and most of them had negligible therapeutic activity, the ignorance so contemptuously referred to by Voltaire could do no great harm in general. The human organism was obviously regarded as a sort of *black box* into which the drug was, as Voltaire said, poured, where it performed its healing function (perhaps), and from which it or part of it was eventually discarded.

Today much more is known about the inner structure of this black box, and about what happens to a chemical substance or drug as it travels from the site of administration into the tissues and organs, and out again. The study of what the organism does to or with a drug, as it pursues its journey through the body, is known as pharmacokinetics.[1]

It is fortunate that we now have a greater knowledge of pharmacokinetics, in view of the highly active but potentially toxic nature of modern drugs. The doctor of today, and tomorrow, must be alert to the many factors that influence the way the body deals with drugs, so that he can, by precisely tailored dosage schemes, produce the desired therapeutic effect.

The introduction of a drug into the body at the site of administration is followed by absorption into the blood stream. Distribution then occurs to various tissues and organs, on some of which the drug may exert its characteristic pharmacological actions. After distribution, the drug begins to make its way out of the body, mainly by excretion into the urine; or it may be chemically altered (metabolized). The metabolite or metabolites may or may not be pharmacologically active, but they are usually more readily excreted into the urine than the original compound. Often, a drug is partly metabolized and partly excreted unchanged.

The variable combination of metabolism and excretion is conveniently referred to as *elimination*, as both processes cause disappearance of the original drug. However, there is no guarantee that one or more of the metabolites may not possess the actions of the parent drug to a greater or lesser degree. These possibilities have to be taken into account by the therapeutician when deciding on the size and frequency of dosage.

In fact, the original drug may have no intrinsic activity of its own, but has to be metabolized to the active substance in the body. This has sometimes not been realized at the outset of a drug's career. Domagk, in 1935, discovered an antibacterial agent which he called Prontosil, chemically a sulphonamide linked with a dyestuff (see p. 23). Actually, Prontosil turned out later to be inactive, and it is the sulphonamide released in the body by metabolic change that attacks the bacteria. The dyestuff was a needless addition to the molecule.

Any drug which is administered so that it finds its way into the blood stream must cross several biological barriers. For example, a drug that is swallowed has to be absorbed through the mucosa (lining) of the stomach or intestine before it can reach the blood vessels. Even a drug injected directly into a vein from the needle of a syringe (intravenous injection) will have to diffuse through the walls of the small capillary blood vessels before it can arrive at the place where it acts, e.g., muscle fibre, nerve cell and so on.

It has been necessary, therefore, for pharmacologists to investigate carefully the factors which determine how well a drug can diffuse across the body barriers. These barriers are composed of layers of cells, which are individually surrounded by membranes containing a high proportion of fatty material known as phospholipid. A drug can in general only pass through these membranes if it has the ability to dissolve in the membrane phospholipid. This means that the capacity of a drug to be rapidly absorbed into the body is related to an important property called lipid solubility.

The lipid solubility of a drug is related to its chemical structure, and is also dependent on the degree to which it is ionized (i.e., split up into positively and negatively charged fragments). The more a drug is ionized in the body fluids, the less lipid soluble it will be, and the less well it will dissolve in, and diffuse through, the cell membrane. Most drugs are either weakly acidic or weakly basic substances, and their degree of ionization depends on the acidity or alkalinity of the fluids in which they are dissolved. A weak acid ionizes better in an alkaline solution, but hardly ionizes at all in a strongly acid medium. Exactly the opposite is true of a drug which is a weak base.

In parenthesis, it should be noted that many naturally occurring substances in the body, e.g., essential nutrients and hormones, can pass through cell membranes by special processes. In facilitated diffusion, the substance is transported passively by means of a carrier from one side of the membrane to the other. In active transport, the substance is transferred by processes that require metabolic energy. Some drugs, presumably for reasons related to their chemical structure, can become involved in these processes. Active transport characteristically occurs through nerve membranes, the choroid plexus of the brain, the tubular cells of the kidney and hepatocytes (liver cells). For example, an active mechanism transports penicillin out of the cerebrospinal fluid of the brain back to the blood (see p. 85).

An understanding of lipid solubility, and its relationship to ionization, is helpful to the practising doctor. Take, for example, aspirin which, as its chemical name acetylsalicylic acid reveals, is a quite strongly acidic substance. After a tablet of this drug is swallowed, it dissolves in the gastric juice which is strongly acid. The acid medium of the stomach will suppress the ionization of the aspirin molecule and so increase its lipid solubility. The drug will, therefore, diffuse rapidly through the stomach mucosa into the blood stream, and from there reach the brain and other tissues to exert its actions.

It is common experience that the actions of aspirin begin quite soon after swallowing the drug. Suppose a person has taken many tablets in an attempt to commit suicide. It could be life-saving to remove as much of the drug as possible by stomach pump (gastric lavage), and then to introduce activated charcoal into the stomach to absorb as much as possible of what aspirin remains there. Many years ago, a common method was to leave behind after gastric lavage a strong alkaline solution of sodium bicarbonate. The sodium bicarbonate was supposed to neutralize the remaining gastric hydrochloric acid and, by making the stomach contents alkaline, promote the ionization of the residual aspirin. This ionized aspirin would then be poorly absorbed into the circulation.

This strategy turned out to be disappointing, since it is difficult to render the stomach contents alkaline in this way, and charcoal worked better. However, it is still customary to make the urine more alkaline by infusion of sodium bicarbonate, thereby promoting the urinary excretion of absorbed aspirin by similar actions on its ionization.

Some drugs are so strongly ionized in body fluids that it is pointless giving them by mouth at all; the molecules are too lipid insoluble to be absorbed. It is necessary to inject them, e.g., into the vascular muscle (intramuscular) where the barriers to absorption are easier to overcome, or better still, directly into a vein (intravenous). This is unwelcome news to the patient, who usually prefers to take his tablets home to ingest at his convenience, so long as they do not taste too nasty and are of a shape and size easy to swallow.

There are other reasons why some drugs are useless if taken by mouth. A swallowed drug is exposed to the potentially destructive actions of the acid in the stomach and of the digestive enzymes. The earliest penicillin (benzylpenicillin), for example, had to be injected because it is readily destroyed by gastric acid.

Even if the drug does manage to cross the gut mucosa unchanged, it will be transported immediately to the liver where it may be broken down by that organ's metabolizing enzymes (the so-called first pass effect). Nitroglycerine, given to relieve the severe pains of angina pectoris, would be inert if swallowed because of almost complete destruction in the liver. This means that hardly any drug would get to the general circulation and to the heart where it is needed. The problem is neatly circumvented by crushing the tablet of nitroglycerin in the mouth, and placing the fragments under the tongue (sublingual administration). Absorption from this site into the blood stream is rapid and reliable, mainly because the substance is very lipid soluble; and its arrival at the liver is delayed for anatomical reasons.

Other mucosal surfaces, as well as those of the tongue, stomach and small intestine, can be utilized for drug absorption. Cocaine addicts and snuff-takers sniff the drug up their noses; absorption from the nasal mucosa is efficient but uncomfortable. The analgesic drug fentanyl is sometimes administered to children by this route.[2] The rectal mucosa can be used for drugs in solution (enemas), or in solid form (suppositories). Some misunderstanding by the layman of the mechanisms involved was suggested by a survey in the UK, which revealed that a substantial proportion of patients failed to remove the wrapper before inserting a suppository! Even the skin is permeable to some drugs, and nicotine may be applied in skin patches for those attempting to quit smoking.

Another useful and simple way of giving a solid drug, which has become popular in recent years, is in the form of an aerosol spray. If the particles of the drug are small enough (less than one-thousandth of a millimeter in diameter), and the spray is directed to the back of the throat, rapid and efficient absorption will occur in the lungs. Some drugs for treating bronchial asthma, e.g., adrenaline, isoprenaline, albuterol, can be administered in this way, but care has to be taken not to be over-enthusiastic in their application or overdosage easily occurs. The antidiuretic hormone (ADH) from the pituitary can also be given in this way, and also recently developed preparations of insulin. If the latter proves to be satisfactory, it could relieve diabetic patients of the constant use of the needle.[3]

Drugs given from a syringe are said to be administered by parenteral injection. This has to be done, as a rule, by a medical practitioner or trained nurse, with a sterilized syringe and needle and precautions against sepsis. Heroin addicts who mainline the drug, i.e., inject it into a vein, are notorious for using dirty syringes. They may then get abscesses at the site of injection, and run the risk of septicaemia, AIDS, or Hepatitis B and C transmitted from previous users of the equipment.

Patient preference for oral administration has led the pharmaceutical industry to seek ingenious ways of overcoming those factors which destroy the drug by that route. Drugs sensitive to gastric acid are enclosed in capsules of gelatin or other resistant materials which do not dissolve until they reach the duodenum and small intestine, where the environment is alkaline or neutral. These preparations are known as enteric-coated drugs.

In general, efficiency of absorption is improved by applying drugs to a larger area with a generous blood flow, e.g., the alveolar epithelium of the lungs that absorbs general anaesthetic drugs so rapidly, and nitroglycerine to the sublingual area.

If absorption by oral and parenteral administration were both effective, then the decision about which route to select would depend on the rate of absorption desired. In general, intravenous injection of a drug leads to the fastest onset of therapeutic action, and is often mandatory in a medical emergency. Oral administration gives the slowest rate of absorption as a rule. Intramuscular injections are rather slower than intravenous, but faster than subcutaneous ones because of the greater blood supply of muscle. Subcutaneous injections are given by introducing the injecting needle just under the skin.

Some special forms of injection are useful when the physician tries to imitate the slow and continuous release into the circulation of the minute amounts of a hormone produced by an endocrine gland. One method is to use plastic coated pills with a minute pore through which the drug is released slowly, or pills which take up tissue fluid so that the pressure inside rises and the drug is forced out at a constant rate. The replacement drug can also be compressed into solid pellets which are implanted under the skin, e.g., subcutaneous implants of corticosteroids or sex hormones. The drug diffuses very slowly into the body fluids, and the therapeutic action may last for several months before a new implant is needed. The problem in replacement therapy, of course, is to mimic the precisely regulated release of a natural hormone according to metabolic requirements. These regulating processes depend on complex feedback mechanisms between endocrine glands and centres in the brain.

To devise methods of drug administration in which the release of an agent is monitored according to need is at the moment the medical inventor's dream, but progress is being made. Small electric pumps, either implanted or attached externally, can infuse the required dose of an analgesic to treat chronic pain. One day we shall be able to make a small, battery-powered intravenous injection kit, incorporating sensor elements which can respond instantaneously to the physiological state of the patient by altering the infusion rate. This sort of device would be invaluable, for example, in the insulin treatment of diabetes mellitus, and in fact progress is already being made towards this goal.

12

Pharmacokinetic Principles

To obtain the right effect at the right intensity, at
the right time, for the right duration, with minimum
risk of harm is what pharmacokinetics is about.

D.R. Laurence and P.N. Bennett,
Clinical Pharmacology (1980)

Following administration and absorption into the circulation (described in
the last chapter), drugs are usually distributed widely throughout body
fluids and tissues. The rate at which they do this depends largely on the
properties of the drug molecules, and how well they penetrate certain
regions of the body such as the brain.

In some cases, however, a substance introduced into the blood stream
may remain there, or at any rate diffuse out into the tissues very slowly. On
occasion, this can be exploited. For example, certain synthetic polymers
known as dextrans have molecules too big to escape through the
capillaries, and solutions of dextran (e.g., Dextran 40 Injection or Dextran
70 Injection) can be given intravenously as plasma substitutes for
emergency transfusions when supplies of blood are not immediately
available.

If a drug binds strongly to proteins in the blood plasma, then the drug-
protein complex will also be too large to diffuse out of the circulation. This
complex will dissociate to release small amounts of the free drug according
to an equilibrium depending on the strength of binding. Only the free,
unbound drug can exert pharmacological actions and the complex is
inactive. Drugs combined with plasma proteins remain much longer in the
body, and the complex acts as a store or reservoir of free drug which is

released in small quantities to find its way out of the circulation to act on the appropriate tissues.

This situation can give rise to an unexpected type of drug interaction. A patient is given drug A which is bound to plasma protein (usually the albumin fraction). The binding equilibrium is such that a small proportion of the drug (say 10%) is in the free, unbound state. This free drug concentration is sufficient to provide a therapeutic effect as a result of the ordinary processes of distribution. If another drug B is now administered which binds even more firmly to the albumin, this will displace by competition appreciable amounts of the drug A. The levels of the free drug A will now increase, and may reach into the toxic range for that drug.

This happens with the antiepileptic drug phenytoin, which is extensively bound (about 90%) to plasma proteins, mainly albumin. If a patient on phenytoin is subsequently given the antidiabetic drug tolbutamide or salicylates, these somewhat stronger protein-binding drugs may displace phenytoin to increase the free, active levels of that drug. The effect is not great, however. A more marked effect is shown by valproate (also antiepileptic) or phenylbutazone (antirheumatic) which reduce both the protein-binding and liver metabolism of phenytoin. In the newborn, displacement of the unconjugated bile pigment bilirubin by sulphonamides may increase the risk of brain damage (encephalopathy) by the bilirubin.

The penetration of drugs into the brain is an essential feature of many so-called centrally acting agents, e.g., anaesthetics, analgesics, hypnotics, sedatives, and tranquillizers. There are, however, some mysteries about this apparently simple process. Since the brain receives about 16% of the volume of blood pumped out by the heart, it is clear that a high proportion (nearly one-sixth) of any drug present in the circulation arrives at the brain. But whether the drug will actually pass through the various barriers to act on vital brain centres is another matter altogether.

As with membranes elsewhere in the body, easy penetration by a drug is directly related to its lipid solubility. The barbiturate thiopentone (Pentothal), which is used as a short-acting intravenous anaesthetic in minor surgery, crosses into the brain rapidly because of its exceptionally high lipid solubility. Anaesthesia comes on almost immediately, as anyone who has had such an injection can testify; but, for the same reasons, when the injection is stopped and the blood thiopentone concentration begins to fall, the drug diffuses equally rapidly out of the brain to restore equilibrium, and anaesthesia promptly ceases. This is also true of many of the gaseous or volatile anaesthetics used in major surgery. Due to their high lipid solubility, they can leave the brain by a process of rapid diffusion.

On the other hand, drugs which are less lipid soluble, and especially those which are ionized in body fluids, appear to have somewhat greater difficulty in crossing barriers in the brain than those in other organs. The slower diffusion of these substances to neurons and other target cells in the central nervous system is believed to be partly due to the unique properties of the epithelial cells of the brain capillaries. These have no intercellular pores, so aqueous flow is severely restricted. The neuroglial cells surrounding the capillaries are also thought to contribute to the slow diffusion of organic acids and bases into the central nervous system. However, the complete mechanisms involved are still probably not fully understood, and we cover our ignorance by talking of the blood-brain barrier.[1] It seems likely that many properties of the blood-brain barrier are derived from protective mechanisms developed during evolution to prevent damage to the central nervous system by toxic substances generated by normal body metabolism. One such device, for example, can actively push unwanted substances back into the blood stream as soon as they penetrate the brain membranes. These substances, therefore, have no chance to exert their toxicity on the brain.

Drugs may find themselves caught up in these active processes of rejection by the brain; one example is penicillin which is a fairly acidic substance. It is no good giving it by parenteral injection for the treatment of cerebral infections, because it penetrates poorly into the brain, or, more accurately, it is immediately transported out again as soon as it gets in. For cerebral infections it would be necessary to give the antibiotic carefully and directly into the cerebro-spinal fluid (the fluid surrounding the brain tissues). Too much penicillin given by this route, however, can cause seizures. Of course, if one gave a sufficiently large dose of the antibiotic parenterally, enough could penetrate into the brain with similar adverse effects.

Another drug transfer which is not fully understood is that across the placenta from the maternal circulation to that of the growing foetus. Again, lipid soluble substances diffuse very readily across the placenta in both directions, but more ionizable compounds may not diffuse quite so efficiently. However, there does not seem to be any form of placental barrier akin to the blood-brain barrier. On the other hand, the placenta is a chemically active tissue rich in enzymes, and drugs may be converted there to toxic metabolites which then reach the foetus. This is thought to be what happened with thalidomide. Unfortunately, the immature liver of the foetus is incompetent when it comes to destroying these toxic metabolites. All doctors should, therefore, be extremely cautious in administering drugs of any kind to a woman who is pregnant, especially during the first three months of gestation when developing tissues are being combined into functional organs (the so-called period of organogenesis).

Some drugs after distribution throughout the body are then selectively concentrated in certain tissues, and this process is known as re-distribution. For example, once thiopentone has left the brain, it eventually finds its way to adipose tissue where it remains for many hours. This is due, of course, to the very high fat solubility of the drug. The insecticide chlorophenothane (DDT) is also stored in fatty tissues for the same reason (see Chap. 15, p. 105).

Bones actively take up calcium from the blood, especially during the growing years of life, and certain elements, like strontium and lead which are chemically similar to calcium, may compete with this mechanism. Strontium is present as the radioactive isotope strontium-90 in the fall-out from atmospheric nuclear explosions. After seven years, only about one-half of this radio-strontium will have decayed or been removed from the body by excretion.

Because of the exceedingly slow clearance of lead stored in bones, one needs to ingest only infinitesimal quantities of the metal over a long period to accumulate considerable amounts in the body. This effect is known as cumulative toxicity. For example, a polluted water supply containing two parts per million of lead will eventually cause toxicity in those who drink it, and since more than 98% of the air pollution in smog-ridden cities is said to be derived from automobile exhaust fumes, the use of leaded gasoline may also lead to chronic poisoning. Owing to the insidious onset of symptoms, cumulative toxicity may be very difficult to diagnose. (See Chap. 14, p. 101 for a fuller account of environmental lead poisoning.)

Strontium-90 and lead present toxicological rather than pharmacological problems. Some drugs, however, can combine with calcium, and the complex is then incorporated into bony tissues. The antibiotics of the tetracycline group are taken up in this way, and it is the effect on developing teeth which is important here. Infants and young children are particularly susceptible; the teeth may show defective enamel, pitting, yellow or brown pigmentation and increased liability to decay. After the fourteenth week of pregnancy and in the first few months of infancy, even short courses of tetracycline can damage developing teeth.

Taken up to the age of four, tetracycline may affect the permanent front teeth, and to avoid adverse effects in all permanent teeth (including wisdom teeth) these drugs should ideally be avoided up to the age of 12.

There are other unexpected drug destinations. Drugs can appear in the saliva or sweat, possibly causing disagreeable tastes or odours; or in the breast milk, from which a nursing mother may transfer dangerous drugs to her infant. It is, in general, the more lipid soluble drugs which turn up in these fluids and secretions.

The elimination of a drug from the body occurs in two ways: by chemical change (metabolism) to another substance or to other substances; and by excretion, mainly in the urine. Some aspects of drug metabolism have been touched upon in previous chapters, and only excretion will be discussed here.

The kidneys are the most important route by which the body rids itself of drugs and their metabolites, but the mechanisms of urinary excretion are quite complicated. The fluid formed in those filtering structures of the kidney, known as glomeruli, contains all components of the blood plasma except the high molecular weight proteins. This filtrate will, of course, include all drugs in the blood stream *except* those that are strongly bound to plasma proteins.

The filtrate then trickles down a complex tubular system from which substances important to the body economy (e.g., glucose, aminoacids) are actively reabsorbed into the circulation. Across these tubular membranes lipid soluble drugs can also passively diffuse back into the body, and this will prolong their duration of pharmacological activity. More ionizable drugs, on the other hand, will tend to remain in the filtrate and not be reabsorbed. This explains why the metabolites of drugs, which are usually less lipid soluble than the original drug, are more readily excreted in the urine.

Drugs which are quite strong acids or bases may be actively pushed in the opposite direction, from blood stream to glomerular filtrate through the tubular membranes. This active process of excretion occurs with penicillin, and is an important reason why the antibiotic stays for only an hour or so in the body after administration.

It is clear from even this brief sketch of the principles of pharmacokinetics that what happens to a drug as it moves into, around, and out of the body can be a very complicated story indeed, and really requires expression in mathematical terms for complete understanding. The mathematical constant which is probably of most practical use to a physician is the *biological half-life* of a drug; or the time taken for elimination of 50% of a single dose from the body. (The reason for choosing 50% is that theoretically there is never, in most cases, complete or 100% elimination. An analogy is the rate of decay of a radioactive element, which is proportional to the amount remaining, and so complete disappearance is never achieved.)

Drugs with a long half-life ($t_{1/2}$), e.g., digoxin (48 hours), need only be administered infrequently, say once a day. A drug which has a short half-life, e.g., penicillin (30 minutes), requires more frequent dosage. A knowledge of the biological half-life, or $t_{1/2}$, is essential, therefore, in deciding the most effective dosage schedule for a given drug.

13

How Drugs Act

First Doctor: ... Domandabo causam et rationem
Quare opium facit slumberum.

Candidate: ... To which respondeo
(Argan) Quia est in eo
Virtus dormitiva,
Cujus est natura
Sensus to soothum.

Chorus of Bene, bene, bene, bene respondere,
Examining Dignus, dignus he to enter
Doctors: Into our docto corpore;
Bene, bene respondere!

Molière (1622–73), translated by K.P. Wormely,
Le Malade Imaginaire, "Epilogue (The Ceremony)"

An exact knowledge of the movements of a drug in and out of the body is, as we have seen, important to the physician who plans an effective dosage schedule. Of greater interest to the patient, perhaps, is an assurance that during these wanderings the drug will produce on some cell, tissue or organ, a desired pharmacological or therapeutic effect. The study of how drugs actually bring about their actions is known as *pharmacodynamics.*[1] To express it in simple terms, whereas pharmacokinetics considers what the body does to or with a drug, pharmacodynamics deals with what the drug does to the body, i.e., its mode or mechanism of action.

The mode of action of many drugs is no longer quite so mysterious today as it was to the primitive medicine man or shaman who concocted his traditional herbal mixtures, and invoked the healing power of the gods. In mediaeval times, medical students chanted parrot-fashion in Latin that opium induced sleep "quia est in eo virtus dormitiva" (because there is in it a soporific virtue). No one could deny this, but the concept is sterile and unhelpful. Molière, in the seventeenth century, used these words to raise a laugh at the end of his comedy *Le Malade Imaginaire*, in which he parodied the medical profession's love of pretentious pseudo-Latin to confuse and impress the laity.

Today, with the development of structural organic chemistry and cell biology, we have learned to visualize a drug's action as the outcome of physico-chemical interactions between that drug and functionally important regions in the living cell known as receptors. The *virtus dormitiva* of opium's main active constituent morphine has, so to speak, been narrowed down to the cellular and subcellular levels. Recent research has revealed a great deal about the fine details of these drug-receptor interactions, though much remains to be clarified. We have to admit that we still lack a profound understanding of how these interactions can actually cause pain relief, sleep, anaesthesia, and so on.

The first approach to the problem of the drug-receptor interaction is to determine the chemical structure of the drug molecule itself; and modern techniques of three-dimensional imaging give us further information about the shape and location of the active chemical groupings in that molecule. We can then identify those parts of the drug molecule which will fit snugly into complementary sites on the receptor molecule. A helpful analogy is that of lock and key. The right active drug (key) applied to the receptor (lock) will modify its configuration (open the lock), and start the macromolecular chain reaction. This leads to the concept of structure-activity relationship (SAR), which opens up the possibility of synthesizing new compounds with similar active groups, and these may be better drugs than the original. The structure and stereochemistry of the receptor sites have also been investigated using three-dimensional imaging. Progress has been slow, but we are beginning to understand more clearly exactly what happens there (see later in this chapter).

One very striking feature of many drugs and toxins, no doubt recognized vaguely by primitive man, is their staggering potency. Minute amounts may cause powerful disorganization of bodily function, even to the point of death. This became yet more obvious when chemists were able to purify the active constituents of medicinal herbs.

The toxin from a bacterium *Clostridium botulinus* will kill a mouse at a dose of one million-millionth of a gram (one picogram). Some natural hormones produce their specific effects at extraordinarily low doses. Ten nanograms (ten thousand-millionths of a gram) of antidiuretic hormone from the pituitary gland can influence kidney function. The therapeutic dose of Vitamin B12 is about one microgram (one millionth of a gram). Pharmacologists studying the actions of substances on isolated animal tissues (e.g., intestine, heart) have elicited responses with quantities of the order of nanograms or even picograms. However, infinitesimal amounts like these still contain many millions of individual molecules.

In 1953, an English Professor of Materia Medica at Edinburgh University, A.J. Clark,[2] made a rough but illuminating calculation. He determined the minimum concentration of a drug strophanthin, which could produce a physiological response on the isolated heart of a frog. Knowing the number of strophanthin molecules in his solution and the approximate number of cells in a frog heart, he estimated the number of drug molecules fixed to each heart cell. The figure came to ten million, which sounds a lot. But further simple arithmetic indicated that even all these molecules could cover only 2–3% of the total surface of a single heart cell. A.J. Clark concluded: "The simplest possible conception of drug action is that potent drugs occupy certain specific areas on the cell surface, and that these specific areas comprise only a small fraction of the total cell surface." These specific areas are the receptors, and receptor theory is one of the corner-stones of modern pharmacodynamics.

Most receptors are now known to be protein macromolecules embedded in the cell membrane for which the active drug has a special affinity. As mentioned above, the active group or groups in the drug molecule fit into a cleft or cavity in this receptor protein. The attachment can be imagined as stretching or distorting the receptor molecule so as to produce changes in the physiological machinery of the cell which alter its functional activity. Many types of such change have been demonstrated, e. g., the opening of channels to facilitate the flow in and out of the cell of certain physiologically active ions like sodium (Na^+), potassium (K^+) or calcium (Ca^{++}). These ion-selective channels are typically acted on by neurotransmitters, leading to alteration in the cell's electrical membrane potential (e.g., the nicotinic cholinergic receptor, see Chap. 17, p. 124). Other types of change are possible, e.g., receptor activation may initiate a chain reaction via other linked proteins in the cell. This can occur because receptors may have two functional sites, the ligand binding (recognition) site or domain where the drug attaches, and an effector (signalling) domain which creates actions via other molecules (e.g., the so-called second messengers).

However, in spite of the complex interactions described above, drugs do not actually cause their pharmacological actions, but merely modulate the intrinsic functions of the receptors on which they act. Receptors can, in fact, be regarded as catalysts, and hence as biochemical signal amplifiers.

There are, indeed, some analogies between receptors and enzymes, both are biological catalysts. With enzymes, it is the substrate molecule attached to it whose chemical bonds are stretched and deformed, leading to its modification or break-up. In fact, some receptors also act as enzymes, e. g., as protein kinases which bind peptide hormones that regulate growth, development and metabolic activity.

For these reasons, investigators have examined the properties of receptors using the techniques by which biochemists have studied isolated enzymes for many years. Some receptors have been removed from the cell membrane or cloned, and their properties submitted to modern techniques, e.g., radioligand assays to demonstrate specific drug binding, microiontophoresis, and patch clamping.[3] There is a problem, however. Once the receptors have been removed from the cell membrane and the specific drugs have been shown to combine with them, one can no longer study the cellular actions they would produce *in situ* because they are detached from their functional chain of proteins in the cell.

We must now consider an important implication of the receptor theory. Receptors were obviously not evolved to combine with the constituents of herbs or the synthetic artefacts of the laboratory. If a substance made by a poppy plant can numb pain by some action on a receptor in a brain cell, then that receptor must possess a function which antedates the acquaintance of man with morphine.

In fact, we know that the ordered growth and the coordinated functioning of any multicellular organism have to be regulated by a whole series of chemical messengers produced by the organism itself. The mechanism is incredibly ingenious in that these messengers can unlock only one type of receptor, and this explains the extraordinary specificity of the process. Many hormones, for example, are released from the pituitary gland into the general circulation, but each stimulates only one organ or tissue in the body, i.e., it unlocks the receptors in one target organ only. If a drug acts on a cell receptor to produce the same effects as the natural messenger, then it must possess some chemical or structural similarity to the messenger so that it can bind to the receptor and initiate the necessary configurational changes.

Such a drug is called an agonist, and the body's messengers are usually described as hormones or transmitters. Morphine, for example, is an analgesic because it can imitate the actions of certain naturally occurring substances in the brain, the enkephalins. More than 40 years ago, the physiologist Hans Kosterlitz, working at the University of Aberdeen, Scotland, was pondering the curious question: how on earth could a chemical substance present in poppies act so effectively to produce analgesia in animals? One possible mechanism would be some alteration in the levels or balance of certain neurotransmitters in the brain (see Part II for a fuller discussion of brain transmitters). Kosterlitz was possibly the first to speculate that the brain itself manufactured a natural chemical with morphine-like properties. After ten years of intensive research, Kosterlitz and his associates isolated from pig brains a substance or substances with just those properties. These compounds came to be known as enkephalins, and later as endorphins. They turned out, not surprisingly, to be quite dissimilar chemically to morphine itself; they were, in fact, pentapeptides (five aminoacids combined in a specific sequence).[4]

However, there must be something common to the molecular configurations of morphine and the enkephalins which enables them to act effectively on pain receptors in the brain.

Drugs are not always merely agonists, and the receptor theory can help us understand some other modes of action. If a drug binds strongly to a receptor, but fails to promote the right configurational change, then it will act as an antagonist to the natural messenger. The key fits, but jams the lock. The drug naltrexone is useful for antagonizing the actions of morphine. It binds more strongly to the enkephalin receptors than the agonist morphine, but produces no action. If morphine is already bound to the receptors, the naltrexone displaces it by competition and so effectively reverses the actions of the morphine.

Certain drugs are known as partial agonists because they bind to the receptors to produce an action, but one much weaker than that of the true agonist. The key fits, but only half opens the lock. This happens with an old drug nalorphine which has weak morphine-like activity and binds strongly to the receptors. Nalorphine was also once used as an antidote to morphine overdosage, since it can displace the morphine from the receptors, but is obviously not as effective as the pure antagonist naltrexone. A new category of agents are called negative antagonists or inverse agonists.

These stabilize the receptor and prevent it from undergoing the conformational changes normally produced by the agonist.

Receptors themselves also come in a variety of subtypes, and this is relevant when deciding on a choice of agonist or antagonist for specific therapeutic purposes. This distinction dates back to the early work of Sir Henry Dale on the cholinergic receptors (see Chap. 17, p. 124). He realized that acetylcholine receptors exist in two forms, serving different physiological functions. One type, which he called muscarinic, is stimulated by muscarine and blocked by atropine. The other type, the nicotinic, is stimulated (initially) by nicotine and blocked by ganglionic blockers such as tubocurarine. Since that time, multiple subtypes of practically all receptors have been identified, usually as a result of a study of the effects of specific agonists and antagonists.

For example, the natural transmitter for all receptors of the sympathetic nervous system (see Chap. 19, p. 133) is noradrenaline, but these have been differentiated into at least two alpha-receptors (α_1 and α_2) and three beta-receptors (β_1, β_2 and β_3). They can be distinguished because each receptor type has its own specific drug agonists and antagonists. For example, β_1- and β_2-receptors control the activity of two kinds of muscle (respectively the smooth muscle of blood vessels, and other smooth muscle and skeletal muscle). β_3-receptors control lipolysis (fat metabolism) in adipose tissue. Receptors for the substance histamine are of two types: H_1 which regulate the microcirculation, and H_2 which are involved in the secretion of hydrochloric acid in the stomach. There are also a wide range of morphine receptors (enkephalin receptors) μ_1, μ_2, κ_1, κ_2, κ_3 and δ.

These distinctions are important in therapeutics because it then becomes possible to design synthetic agonists, antagonists and partial agonists more or less specific for a particular receptor subtype. H_1-receptor antagonists (mepyramine) can be useful in relieving histamine-induced bronchial constriction and allergic reactions, but do not block gastric acid secretion. H_2-receptor antagonists (e.g., Tagamet) are specific for reducing stomach acid. This therapeutic strategy is likely to reduce dangerous side effects caused by actions on other receptor subtypes.

It should be realized that some drugs are only indirectly involved with receptors, or not involved at all. One obvious example is the direct chemical neutralization of stomach acid by oral antacids (e.g., aluminium hydroxide; Amphogel and many others). Natural hormones and transmitters are often rapidly broken down in the tissues by special enzymes, a process which is an intrinsic part of their functioning. If a drug combines with such a destroying enzyme (*not* the receptor in this case) and inactivates it, then the natural messenger is preserved and may continue to act on its receptors. Such a drug will produce its pharmacological actions by prolonging the activity of the messenger, rather than by any direct effect. Some drugs whose chemical structures are similar to those of important naturally occurring substances in the body may become incorporated into the cellular components, a process known as counterfeit incorporation mechanism. Certain analogues of pyrimidines and purines may be falsely incorporated into nucleic acids, thereby disrupting abnormal (and normal) cell division. These have proved useful in cancer chemotherapy and antiviral treatment (e.g., fluorouracil and Efudex).

In addition, there are drugs which can release stores of a chemical messenger in the tissues, or act on enzymes to promote or decrease the tissue synthesis of these messengers. The overall result is to cause potentiation or inhibition, as the case may be, of the actions of the natural messengers at their receptor sites.

In Part II, we shall quote some examples of drugs used in modern medicine which are believed to act by one or the other of the mechanisms described above.

14

Death in the Environment: Antiquity

> The people of the city said to Elisha, "You can see
> how pleasantly our city is situated, but the water is
> polluted and the country is troubled with miscarriages."
>
> *The New English Bible*, II Kings, 2, v. 19

So far we have limited ourselves almost entirely to the misfortunes inflicted on us by the medical profession when it uses chemical substances to produce possible therapeutic effects. Doctors, however, are not the only purveyors of toxic agents to man. Apart from Nature herself, civilization and industry are other important sources of poisons, some of which we shall consider briefly in the next two chapters. It must be remembered that all that has been said about drugs — their absorption and fate in the human body, and the ways in which they act on organs and tissues — applies equally to those toxic chemicals that appear, for one reason or another, in our immediate environment and poison the general population.[1]

Prehistoric man probably lived in a relatively unpolluted world, though his life was usually *nasty, brutish and short*[2] from disease, tribal conflict, wild animals and natural disasters. He had experience of the poisonous nature of some plants, fruits and fungi, and the occasionally fatal venoms of certain snakes and insects. Many of these natural poisons became, of course, components of primitive pharmacopoeias (see "Introduction").

Village settlements based on agriculture began to appear between 8,000 and 4,500 B.C. in the mesolithic period with the domestication of plants and animals. These were typically in the hillier regions of the Middle East. Similar communities probably arose independently elsewhere, e.g., in the monsoon areas of Asia, the Pacific Islands and in pre-Columbian America. There was the cultivation of a variety of grains (rye, barley, millet, wheat, and rice) as well as root crops, and it became necessary to harvest and store these for the winter months, together with certain nuts and other edible seeds. Earthenware vessels, fired in primitive kilns and sometimes glazed, were utilized for storage and cooking of these foodstuffs.

The spread of neolithic agricultural and village life overlapped the rise of urban civilizations soon after 4,000 B.C. These appeared in the great river valleys of the Tigris-Euphrates, Nile and Indus, stimulated by the development of irrigation and technology. In particular, in these cities (e. g., Babylon, Memphis, and Mohenjo-Daro), the mining of minerals and the refining of metals became increasingly important. Some of these minerals were used for the glazing of pottery, and occasionally for medicinal purposes, and many, of course, were poisonous.

Under certain climatic conditions the staple foods of these early villagers were attacked, either in the field or during storage, by microfungi (moulds), some species of which produced toxic substances known as mycotoxins. *Aspergillus flavus* may grow on stored corn, nuts, oil seeds (e. g., groundnuts), and produce toxins called aflatoxins. These aflatoxins can cause cancer of the liver in laboratory rats, and may be responsible for the high prevalence of human liver cancer in certain parts of Africa. More important, historically, are the microfungi which infect staple food grains. The toxins they produce may persist in the bread made from these grains, and cause widespread death, especially among infants and children. Some of these mycotoxins also act on the central nervous system (CNS) and alter the behaviour of those ingesting them, leading to mass psychosis in communities and even whole regions. Microfungal poisoning was probably not common in the drier climates of the Near and Middle East, but flourished where agriculture spread to the cooler, wetter climates of Northern Europe. The optimal conditions for microfungal infections were a cool winter which slowed growth of the host grain, followed by a warm, wet summer which favoured parasitic attack. Outbreaks of poisoning from these agents have persisted until quite recent times, and some believe that they may have had a significant influence on historical events in Europe and North America.

The most important of these toxic microfungi is *Claviceps purpurea* which grows on the widely cultivated rye (*Secale cereale*). Spores are carried by the wind or by insects to the rye plant in spring or early summer, and the germinated fungus penetrates deep into the ovary of the grain and eventually replaces it with a hard purplish-black body, technically known as a *sclerotium* or more popularly as the *ergot of rye*. (Ergot is derived from the old French word *argot*, meaning a spur; the sclerotium is a spur-shaped body.) The toxic nature of ergot was probably first recognized by the Assyrians around 600 B.C. They recorded the existence of "a noxious pustule in the ear of grain". Two hundred years later, the Persians wrote: "Among the evil things created … are noxious grasses that cause pregnant women to drop womb and die in childbed." The toxic effects of ergot are now known as ergotism.

It was not until the middle of the seventeenth century in Europe that it was realized that ergot-infected rye was probably responsible for many destructive epidemics of mass poisoning reported from the Middle Ages onwards. The commonest symptoms were vascular changes in the limb extremities which shrivelled, became black and gangrenous and eventually dropped off. The excruciating pain involved was known as Holy Fire (*Ignis Sacer*), or St. Anthony's Fire, from the name of the shrine in France where a cure was said to be obtained (probably from a change of diet at or *en route* to the shrine). There was also a more acute convulsive form of ergotism involving the central nervous system, causing periodic seizures of the limbs and even the trunk itself.

After the introduction of the potato from the New World in the sixteenth century, rye became less important as a food staple in Europe and ergotism was less commonly seen. However, sporadic outbreaks occurred in Northern Europe and Russia, where rye continued to be cultivated, until well into the twentieth century, e.g., in Russia up to 1945, and in France in 1953 (traced to a baker using infected grain). A related fungus *Claviceps microcephala* also produces similar toxins, and still may infect the staple cereal *bajra* (millet) in Rajasthan, India.

Watery extracts of ergot were used in obstetrics from the sixteenth to seventeenth centuries onwards for hastening childbirth, but by midwives, not physicians. The first physician to use ergot for this purpose was the Frenchman Desgranges who called it *poudre obstétricale*. At the beginning of the nineteenth century, John Stearns in the USA got to know of this powder from an old woman who had emigrated from Eastern Europe, and his account of its use in childbirth marked the introduction of ergot into official medicine. However, the new drug was over-enthusiastically applied, leading to many stillbirths. What had been called *pulvis ad partum* became *pulvis ad mortem*.

The first scientific investigation into the active principles of ergot had to wait until 1906, and was carried out by the chemist George Barger and the eminent pharmacologist Sir Henry Dale. They found ergot to be a treasure trove of pharmacologically active substances, with many different kinds of actions on tissues. Historically, their studies formed one of the most important foundation stones of twentieth century experimental physiology and pharmacology. Ergot contains a number of alkaloids (nitrogen-containing organic bases), which are derivatives of a complex substance known as lysergic acid. One group is sparingly soluble in water and so would not be present significantly in aqueous extracts. One example of this group is ergotamine, which is today still used in the treatment of migraine headaches. The second group is water-soluble, and includes ergometrine, which was the main active principle in the extracts used by midwives to contract the pregnant uterus. In recent times, some synthetic derivatives of lysergic acid have been made by chemists, the most striking being the hallucinogen LSD-25 (lysergic acid combined with diethylamine, see Chap. 22, p. 155).

Ergot — and this was of great interest to Sir Henry Dale — also contains a number of pharmacologically active organic amines (substances made up of carbon, hydrogen, oxygen and nitrogen) such as histamine and tyramine. It also contains acetylcholine, which turned out to be a substance of vital physiological importance in the mammalian nervous system (see Chap. 17, p. 124). Dale shared the 1936 Nobel Prize for Physiology and Medicine with Otto Loewi for their pioneer work on the role of acetylcholine in the chemical transmission of nerve impulses. We can, therefore, trace a historical thread linking the spoilage of grain on mesolithic village settlements, epidemics of mass poisoning in medieval Europe and some of the triumphs of twentieth century pharmacology.

However, the mining of mineral ores by the urban civilizations of the great river valleys probably had more insidious and widespread effects on the health of mankind throughout the ages. One has to consider not only the users of the metals refined from these ores into vessels for domestic purposes, but even more the unfortunate workmen, slaves or convicted criminals responsible for digging them out of the ground. Many metals, metalloids and minerals, e.g., lead, mercury, cadmium, arsenic, and asbestos, are toxic to man, and others have come under suspicion in recent years, e.g., the postulated role of aluminium in Alzheimer's Disease (now discounted).[3] One should not forget, too, that miners are liable to be exposed to dust-laden environments containing silica which can cause chronic lung disease (pneumoconiosis).

One of the best-known historical examples of insidious metal poisoning is that produced by lead. Lead ores were probably the first to be mined. Lead poisoning was recognized in antiquity and has by no means been eliminated from the modern world. Even in early times, lead played an important role in industrial, scientific and military progress, as well as in trade, material comfort and the treatment of disease. Lead is often associated geologically with silver, which was always the more desirable metal for ornamental purposes (and also arsenic), but lead is a readily extracted, low melting and malleable metal with many practical applications.

The principal ore for lead extraction is the ubiquitous galena (lead sulphide or *black lead*), which in remote antiquity was itself used cosmetically as an eye-paint. Quite low temperatures will burn off the sulphur, leaving the molten metal. The oldest known piecě of lead, dating back to 6,500 B.C., was found at Çatel Huyuk in modern Turkey. Tumblers made from lead appeared in Mesopotamian grave sites around 3,500–3,000 B.C. There can be little doubt that lead poisoning may be regarded as one of the earliest occupational diseases of mankind. As mentioned in Chap. 12 (p. 86), lead is taken up and stored in bony tissue and is only very slowly cleared from the body: its half-life is several decades. The metal's main adverse effects are on the red blood cells, causing anaemia; on the peripheral nervous system, leading to *wrist-drop* and sensory loss; and (especially in children) a severe encephalopathy manifesting itself in convulsions and eventual coma.

Lead played an enormous role in the Roman economy, and it is not unreasonable to suppose that chronic lead poisoning was widespread in the population. In fact, many writers have ascribed the decline of the Roman Empire and the mental quirkiness of some of the later emperors to the toxic effects of that metal. The Romans preserved fruits and vegetables with lead salts and cooked their meals in leaden pots. Some lead salts have a sweet taste (lead acetate was once known as *sugar of lead*), and in the absence of sucrose they were prized for their sweetening actions, especially in wine. Worse still, wine was often boiled down in leaden vessels. The Romans were also famous for the sophistication of their plumbing, but unfortunately their widespread use of lead piping must have led to the contamination of their water for drinking and cooking. It is estimated that the Roman economy utilized more than 550 grams of lead per person per year, and that 140,000 workmen per year were exposed to its toxicity during mining and manufacture. From early times to about 500 A.D. the worldwide production of lead was probably about 39 million tons, and even until the beginning of the nineteenth century, lead production exceeded that of all other non-ferrous metals.

In Europe, after the fall of the Roman Empire, lead continued to be widely used industrially, and (perhaps in view of its toxicity!) even in medical treatment. Paracelsus boasted that he could cure 200 diseases with lead in various forms — but we must remember that he did not distinguish lead and mercury. Dentists employed lead for dental fillings up to the seventeenth century in a process known as *plombage*. Our modern fears of mercury poisoning from amalgam fillings seem almost frivolous when one considers the much greater dangers likely from plombage. The expression "death in the pot" became famous in the eighteenth century and was derived from a passage in the Bible (II Kings, 4, v. 40). This referred to the widespread and willful adulteration of food with lead salts and other agents, the storage of food in metal containers, and sometimes the abuse of alcoholic drinks. The use of lead pipes to carry domestic water supplies has continued to the present day, and a truly modern source of lead pollution arises from the addition of lead-containing compounds to petrol.[4] The latter use is most dangerous to children living in the inner cities of the USA and elsewhere, and may be their number one environmental poison, leading to mental retardation and impaired school performance, seizures and cerebral palsy. This is still the case even though legislation since the early 1970s eliminates lead from paint and pipes carrying drinking water, and the use of unleaded petrol in motor vehicles has now been phased out in the US and Europe. The lead was present in the form of lead tetraethyl. Unfortunately, this ban is not universal; in Mexico City, for example, cars are said to pump 20 tonnes of lead into the atmosphere every day.

Lead, and other metals such as cadmium and zinc, are detectable in the snow and ice of Greenland, derived from industrial pollution in the northern hemisphere. It was shown in the late 1960s that the levels of lead there had increased 200-fold since pre-industrial times. It is encouraging that, as a result of the introduction of lead-free fuels in the industrial countries at about that time, the levels of so-called anthropogenic lead were beginning to fall in Greenland snows by 1991.[5]

15

Death in the Environment:
The Twentieth Century

Thirty years ago, one in four Americans was
getting cancer and one in five was dying from it.
Today, one in three Americans gets cancer,
and one in four dies from it.

Dr. Samuel Epstein,
Professor of Occupational and Environmental Health,
University of Illinois

Although toxic pollution can be traced back to antiquity, as we saw in the last chapter, it was the Industrial Revolution of the nineteenth century which enormously amplified the prevalence and dangers of occupational and environmental poisoning. There are two main factors involved: the increase in the scale and productivity of those mining and refining processes inherited from the past, and the development and growth of the synthetic chemical industry.

The first factor led in the twentieth century to some spectacular industrial disasters. Mercury, known to the ancient Egyptians and Chinese, has become widely used in many modern manufacturing processes. Between 1953 and 1960 many fishermen and their family members living near Minamata Bay in Japan developed a bizarre neurological syndrome known as Minamata Disease.[1] A factory close by was found to be dumping mercury-containing effluent into the waters of the bay. Micro-organisms converted the metal into very toxic methyl and ethyl derivatives, which then entered the food chain, ending up eventually in the larger food-fish. There were 121 victims of the disease, of whom 46 died.

The metal cadmium was unknown until 1817, but is now widely used in industry. It accumulates slowly in the body, being concentrated especially in the kidneys, and is a possible cause of raised blood pressure (hypertension). Itai-itai disease[1] in Japan — a severe and often fatal condition presenting as osteomalacia (softening of the bones) — affected 200 victims whose rice fields were irrigated by waste water from a mine, and was traced to excessive amounts of cadmium in the effluent.

The growth of the chemical industry has made available to mankind a plethora of hitherto unknown synthetic compounds (mainly carbon-containing), and this presents a much greater threat to our health. It is estimated that in 1990 there were 8 million known chemical substances, and the number increases by 6,000 every week! The majority of these, of course, would exist only in small amounts on laboratory shelves and would have no widespread use. But those that are utilized in agriculture, industry or in the home clearly represent a potential hazard, both occupationally and environmentally. Admittedly, the body has some protection against foreign substances because it has non-specific liver enzymes which can metabolize them to harmless, excretable products (p. 4). Nevertheless, the massive onslaught of all these new chemicals on modern society is something unprecedented in our evolutionary history, and rightly gives cause for alarm. Nor are the non-industrial countries immune from this menace; they may not make these compounds themselves, but are only too readily persuaded to import them from multinational firms. David Weir and Mark Schapiro in their book *The Circle of Poison* (1981)[2] report that the multinational pesticide manufacturers "have turned the Third World into not only a booming growth market for pesticides, but also a dumping ground." Many of these agents are considered too dangerous for direct use in the USA, yet Americans do not necessarily escape their toxicity. "Pesticide exports create a circle of poison, disabling workers in American chemical plants and later returning to us in the food we import."

The substances most likely to cause serious toxicity are those used on a large scale to increase agricultural yields, and in the processing of foodstuffs. Among the former are fungicides, herbicides, insecticides and rodenticides, and the latter include preservatives, colouring, flavouring and sweetening agents, as well as a miscellany of emulsifiers, stabilizers and anti-oxidants. Some insecticides, in particular, have aroused great concern. Many of these kill by disrupting vital metabolic pathways in insects, and since these pathways are also important in man the compounds can be very toxic to human subjects handling them (e.g., cholinesterase inhibitors, see Chap. 18, p. 131).

One of the first insecticides to be widely used was the chlorinated hydrocarbon chlorophenothane (DDT), which, as mentioned in Chap. 7 (p. 54), is fat-soluble and tends to persist for long periods of time in the adipose tissue. (that is, it has a long half-life). The compound does not appear to be itself harmful to man, but its entry into the food chain, leading to adverse effects on birds of prey such as hawks and eagles, caused it to be almost completely banned in the USA in 1972. These birds accumulated DDT from feeding on small animals, resulting in reproductive problems and endangerment of the species. The compound caused thinning of the shells of their eggs, possibly by increasing estrogen metabolism. Since the banning of DDT, levels of the compound in human adipose tissue have diminished significantly, but there can be a human downside to obviously desirable measures of this kind. In the five years following the DDT ban, 4.5 million more children were estimated to have died from malaria worldwide.[3] A similar increase is likely to have occurred with some other tropical vector-borne diseases like filariasis and bilharzia. It should also be remembered that probably about one quarter of all food grown by man is consumed by pests if they are not controlled or eliminated by pesticides, rodenticides, etc. However, what these poisons might do to the more harmless members of the animal kingdom is another story.

Many of the more recent insecticides such as malathion and parathion belong to the organophosphorus family of compounds, whose main activity is the inhibition of the physiologically important enzyme acetylcholinesterase. Some of the most highly toxic of these to man have been developed as nerve gases in warfare. However, although malathion and parathion are potent insecticides, they are relatively non-toxic in mammals. Compared with DDT, they have much shorter half-lives ($t_{1/2}$), i.e., they do not cumulate in tissues and are rapidly metabolized and excreted. Acute toxicity from these and other modern agricultural poisons, e.g., paraquat, is more likely to occur from rare accidents due to ignorance, incompetence or criminal adulteration. For example, in Singapore in 1959, barley contaminated with parathion killed four children. In Iraq in 1972 seed grain treated with a mercury-containing fungicide, which was eaten instead of being planted, caused over 6,000 cases of poisoning, and 459 victims died. Fifteen children in Peru died after eating food from government-distributed bags originally containing organophosphates.

Similar disasters have also occurred with industrial chemicals as a result of criminal action, inadequate labelling and failure of technical control. One of the most tragic of these took place on 2 December 1984, at a Union Carbide plant in Bhopal, India.[4] Technical carelessness and a disregard for safety regulations caused the escape from a partially buried storage tank of a toxic gas, methyl isocyanate. Prevailing winds carried a yellow fog of the gas to the nearby slums where many of the plant workers lived. The death toll was estimated to be 2,500. Two hundred thousand or more were injured, and the disaster was probably the worst industrial accident in history. The long-term effects, both medical and ecological, are yet to be evaluated.

There are a number of ironic facets to the Bhopal story. Union Carbide opened the plant in 1977 with the encouragement of the Indian government in order to manufacture several pesticides based on methyl isocyanate as an intermediate. One of the best known of these is Sevin, which is regarded as relatively non-toxic for humans and is readily biodegradable. The Indian government has for many years adopted modern agricultural techniques, including the use of pesticides like Sevin, in order to make the subcontinent self-sufficient in food production. This policy was so successful that India became a net grain exporter.

Another aim of the Indian government was to provide as many local jobs as possible, and it did this by requiring the plant to be labour intensive. The plant, therefore, intentionally lacked computerized safety systems, and the supervision of manufacturing processes was left to human intervention. Moreover, the plant, though built on the outskirts of the city, attracted workers whose dwellings naturally mushroomed around the factory itself, in defiance of local regulations.

A somewhat similar disaster took place earlier at a Dow Chemical Company factory in Seveso, near the Italian city of Milan, in July 1977.[5] An explosion released a gas cloud containing a toxic dioxin derivative TCDD (2,3,7,8,-tetrachlorodibenzo-p-dioxin) over the surrounding countryside, affecting man, animals and vegetation over a wide area. Ironically, the factory was not trying to make TCDD; in fact, dioxins are not made anywhere intentionally (except in small quantities as reference substances), since they have no commercial or medical use. Actually, the Seveso plant was manufacturing a trichlorophenol used at the time as an intermediate in the synthesis of the mild bactericidal agent hexa-chlorophene. Unfortunately, during the production of the trichlorophenol very small amounts of TCDD were formed as a contaminant, and larger amounts than usual were formed under the increased temperatures and pressures associated with the explosion. Probably about half a pound of

TCDD contaminated the explosive cloud of trichlorophenol and caustic lime at Seveso.

Of the local population, 500 showed signs of poisoning, and pregnant women were advised to have abortions since TCDD was known to be teratogenic in animal tests. More than 600 domestic animals either died or had to be killed. Since TCDD is chemically very stable and persists in the soil, all crops within 8km south of the factory were burned. Owing to initial confusion about the nature of the toxic material in the cloud, the nearby inhabitants were not evacuated until 2 weeks after the explosion, and are likely to be under medical follow-up for the rest of their lives. A 1989 study indicated an increase in brain tumours, leukemia and other cancers in the local population.[6]

TCDD is only one of 75 possible chlorinated dibenzo-p-dioxin derivatives, which are loosely called dioxins. Dioxins also contaminate certain herbicides manufactured for aerial spraying to defoliate and kill vegetation on or near highways, railroads, powerlines and pipelines. These herbicides are chlorophenoxy compounds, the best known being 2,4-D and 2,4,5-T. They became notorious for their widespread use as a defoliant mixture (Agent Orange) during the Vietnam War. The most obvious toxicity of 2,4,5-T in man is a severe contact dermatitis known as chloracne which attacks the head and upper body, is more disfiguring than ordinary acne, and can persist for many years. Systemically, the substance does not accumulate in mammals since it is actively excreted with a half-life in man of about 24 hours. Nevertheless, in view of the general concern about its long-term toxicity and the presence of dioxin contaminants, Dow Chemical announced its decision to stop manufacturing 2,4,5-T in October 1983.

However, the threat of dioxin toxicity could not be so easily set aside. It soon became clear that dioxins are also produced in a number of other industrial processes in which chlorine is used. Some of these are: (1) pulp and paper bleaching; (2) accidental fires involving chlorinated benzenes and biphenyls; (3) improper disposal of certain chlorinated wastes; and (4) certain methods of wood preserving, oil refining and metal smelting. Although the amounts of dioxins formed are presumably minute, the fact that some are very stable and not readily broken down means that they continue to accumulate in the ecosystem, in the adipose tissues of man and in other species at the top end of the food chain. Moreover, they have been described, especially by environmentalists, as the most poisonous substances known to science.

Here a dilemma arises that has fueled a bitter controversy in the USA between the Environmental Protection Agency and industry on the one hand, and the environmentalists on the other. There is no doubt that TCDD is highly toxic to certain animal species, e.g., hamsters, and monkeys, but the degree of toxicity in humans is debatable. Chloracne definitely occurs in man, but liver damage, digestive disorders, depression of the immune system, spontaneous abortions, and teratogenic and carcinogenic effects, well documented in test animals, have not been confidently associated with human exposure. There are obvious reasons for this. Dioxins have no medical applications, so there are no data based on controlled administration to human subjects. Most human exposures occur under circumstances, e.g., industrial accidents, sporadic spraying of herbicides, and wartime use, that make scientific analysis of the results very difficult, if only because these compounds are always associated with other chemicals and solvents which are likely to possess their own intrinsic toxicities.

It is not easy to steer a rational course between the complacency of industry and its lobbying influences on governmental agencies, and the environmentalists' tendency to exaggerate the dangers, in order to arrive at a reasonable assessment of the truth. A 1979 incident illustrates this point. A tank car containing 19,000 gallons of wood preservative contaminated with about one teaspoon of dioxin sprang a leak near Sturgeon, Mississippi. Sixty-five local citizens sued both the railroad and the Monsanto Chemical Company, claiming to suffer headaches, insomnia and depression from the exposure to dioxin. The railroad settled out of court, but the case against Monsanto went to trial. The jury slapped a $16 million penalty on the firm, in spite of a rider saying that there was no evidence that the plaintiffs had been poisoned by the dioxin. Eventually, an appeal court reversed this judgement in 1991.

The appeal court was no doubt right to do this in the circumstances. In fact, a well-known syndicated columnist went so far as to comment that "fear and anxiety about dioxin have disrupted more lives and done more damage to people than the dioxin itself has ever done." But can we be so sure of this? Experience with the long-term effects of chemicals given medically hardly encourages such complacency, in view of the unexpected toxicities that are sometimes revealed after many years of administration of even the apparently safest of drugs (cf. Chap. 6, p. 47). We must remember, too, that with drugs these surprise effects are more likely to be picked up because administration is controlled and recorded by the patients' physicians. The long-term medical results of pollution, if they exist, are much more difficult to correlate with the haphazard and uncontrolled absorption into the body of what may be a mixture of environmental pollutants. Dr. Samuel Epstein, whose cancer statistics were cited at the beginning of this chapter, continued: "I have no doubt that dioxins must be given some credit for this." The jury is still out, but the Professor could be right.

This chapter has so far considered mainly those toxic substances produced on a large scale during industrial activities and those that are used in agriculture, but, as a postscript, we should briefly mention some dangers specific to today's domestic environment. Of course, many products used in building construction, painting and decorating, cleaning, pest destruction, even food preservatives, flavourings and colourings, etc. are manufactured and may have toxic properties. Nowadays, most large populations in the developed world are served by Poison and Drug Information Centres, which can be telephoned for urgent treatment advice in cases of accidental ingestion of, or exposure to, these agents (not to mention the contents of many bathroom drug cabinets).

Here are just a few examples. Several dangerous gases and fine particles can be unsuspectingly inhaled in the assumed safety of one's home: the odourless, colourless gas carbon monoxide (CO) is present in our domestic gas supply which is, however, doctored with an unpleasant smelling material so that leaks can be readily detected. Carbon monoxide can also be emitted by inadequately ventilated furnaces, and is present in car exhaust where it may build up to toxic levels in the confined space of a garage. The radioactive gas radon, a breakdown product of radium, can accumulate in ill-ventilated houses built with materials containing radium. Long-term exposure to radon can cause lung cancer. Fortunately, this pollutant can be readily tested for. Asbestos, once used as an insulating material in building construction, is harmless so long as it remains undisturbed, but if released during remodelling and breathed in as minute particles, it can lead over time to a serious lung tumour known as mesothelioma. Cigarette smokers expose the rest of the family to the toxic components of their smoke. This phenomenon, known as passive smoking, is now clinically proven to affect the health of the non-smokers, a finding reluctantly accepted by the tobacco industry. Tobacco smoke also contains carbon monoxide.

Another potential route by which poisons enter the home is in the tap water used for drinking and cooking. Certain elements, e.g., lead, arsenic, selenium, can be the villains here. Fluoride has also been intentionally added to urban water supplies at low concentrations in order to improve dental health, a measure initially attacked as a threat to personal freedom by its opponents. There is no doubt that too much fluoride may lead to unsightly mottling of the permanent teeth. This is seen naturally in regions where well water, for geological reasons, contains unduly high levels of fluoride. An unexpected bonus of fluoridation is that it tends to decrease osteoporosis in later life (weakening of the bones causing fractures). It could be argued, however, that the widespread availability today of fluoride-containing toothpaste and gels makes it less important to add this element to tap water.

The problem of lead in tap water from lead pipes has been mentioned in Chap. 12 (p. 86) The presence of arsenic in urban water supplies is also a matter of concern (sometimes over-concern) for many citizens, but there are usually regulations mandating reduction to acceptable levels. Arsenic may be too high in well water derived from areas where the element is abundant in soils, e.g., Argentina, Chile, Taiwan and certain regions of the western US. Like lead, arsenic has a venerable history going back 2,400 years to Greece and Rome, where it was used in therapeutics and for intentional poisoning. These uses continued up to almost modern times, e. g., in the 1880s arsenic (in the form of Paris Green) was a component of some paints and wallpapers, and later of many domestic weedkillers. Its use in modern therapeutics is limited to certain tropical diseases, e.g., trypanosomiasis. Arsenic shows some similarities to lead in that it is slowly excreted from the body ($t_{1/2}$ 3–5 days) and cumulates specifically in keratin-containing tissues like hair and nails. These properties have made arsenic a favourite chronic poison for detective story writers, since the substance can be detected chemically in those tissues, even posthumously and after exhumation of the corpse. Another tell-tale sign is the appearance of transverse white lines of deposited arsenic in the finger nails (Mee's lines) about six weeks after exposure to the element.[7]

Another element, selenium, can also be an environmental pollutant (an important source is the industrial burning of coal) and turn up in drinking water. It is a curious substance which does have a genuine function as an essential trace element in the body. It is a component of an important enzyme glutathione peroxidase, which reduces hydrogen peroxide to water. Selenium may, therefore, facilitate the antioxidant action of Vitamin E. However, it is toxic in large doses, the upper limit in water being ten micrograms per litre. Some claim that it can help prevent cancer, but this remains to be proved. The recommended daily allowance (RDA) is 40 to 70 micrograms for men and 45 to 65 micrograms for women.

Part II

Here was a panacea ... for all human woes; here was the
secret of happiness, about which philosophers had disputed
for so many ages, at once discovered; happiness might now
be bought for a penny, and carried in the waistcoat-pocket;
portable ecstasies might be corked up in a pint-bottle;
and peace of mind could be sent down by the mail.

Thomas de Quincey, in
Confessions of An English Opium Eater (1821)

16

Drugs and the Mind

The services rendered by intoxicating substances
in the struggle for happiness and in warding off
misery rank so highly as a benefit that both
individuals and races have given them an established
position within their libido-economy. It is
not merely the immediate gain in pleasure which
one owes to them, but also a measure of that
independence of the outer world which is so sorely
craved ... We are aware that it is just this
property which constitutes the danger and
injuriousness of intoxicating substances ...

Sigmund Freud, in *Civilization, War and Death* (1939)

Of the many drugs known to us, those which act on the brain to modify our thoughts, feelings, mood and behaviour arouse the most interest and curiosity. Moreover, these psychotropic drugs, as they are now called, have been widely used and abused by mankind throughout its long history.

Aldous Huxley wrote in 1957: "All the naturally occurring sedatives, narcotics, euphoriants, hallucinogens and excitants were discovered thousands of years ago, before the dawn of civilisation ... By the late Stone Age man was systematically poisoning himself ... There were dope addicts before there were farmers." The fact that chemicals out of a bottle or from a growing plant can affect our moods, our behaviour and even our state of consciousness, is quite a challenge to our almighty egos. Since the ego that claims to control each human mind is a part of that mind, the mind itself resents the fact that drugs can disrupt its efficient and supposedly autonomous functioning.

It is not necessary here to embroil ourselves in a philosophical discussion of what exactly the mind is and how it is related to the brain (the so-called mind-body problem). But we can all agree, probably, that the concept of man's mind encompasses collective human knowledge, skills, customs and beliefs, amalgamated with specific individual memories, experiences, moods, temperaments and personality. Clearly, all this is, in some mysterious way, more than the 1.4kg brain which can lie, inactive and irrecoverable, on an anatomist's slab for dissection. Yet what we mean by *mind* must somehow be imprinted, stored or programmed in man's incredibly complex living brain or central nervous system (CNS), and can be actively recalled for introspection or communication to other minds. When drugs affect the mind, they must do so through some action on the CNS itself. First of all, therefore, we have to consider how the physical brain, and in fact the nervous system in general, comes to be vulnerable to the presence of alien chemicals or drugs.

The nervous system in man and other animals comprises more than just the brain. These are the spinal cord and the peripheral motor and sensory nervous systems, as well as the autonomic nervous system (ANS) which controls many of the automatic functions of the body like respiration, blood flow and digestion. The brain itself has connections with the peripheral and autonomic systems, and partially controls and organizes them. It is not mere size of the brain which makes for man's superior intelligence (the porpoise, the elephant and the whale have bigger ones), but its degree of development and complexity of organization. Yet, in spite of this complexity, which has by no means been fully explored and mapped, the structural elements involved are essentially no different from those present in the much simpler brains or nervous systems of lower organisms.

The basic component of all nervous systems is the *neuron*, a specialized cell with a nucleus from which emerge one or more processes or *axons*. Down these axons, which may be long or short, minute electrical currents flow rapidly to the nerve ending which terminates close to a tissue or organ, or to another neuron. The small gap between the nerve ending and the adjacent cell or neuron, measuring only millionths of a millimeter in length, is known as the *synapse*.

Fundamentally, a nerve process can do only two things: it can conduct an electrical impulse or not conduct it. Neurons (there are probably well over ten billion in the cortex of the human brain alone) are arranged and organized into nerve tracts, i.e., bunches of nerve fibres (which may run a considerable distance in the body), centres, relay stations, nuclei and so on. Each of these arrangements of neurons performs some essential neurological function as a result of the transmission of patterns of electrical pulses along the associated axons. Nerve tracts are typically surrounded by sheaths of an insulating material known as myelin. These tend to look pinkish in colour in the fresh brain, or white after fixing in formaldehyde solution. Centres, nuclei, etc., are collections of neurons, which look whitish-yellow when fresh, and grey after fixing due to the absence of myelin. These two kinds of structures, myelinated and non-myelinated, show up as areas of so-called *white matter* and *grey matter* in the nervous system.

Since axons can be likened to the insulated wires in a complicated electrical circuit, there was a fashion at one time to compare the nervous system to a telephone exchange. With the development of the microcomputer, this came to be regarded as a better model of the brain. A computer is also built up from an enormous number of micro-circuits which either conduct a current or not. On this simple basis the computer, like the brain, can perform complex manipulations on data presented to it. This model or analogy falls down, unfortunately, in at least one important respect. Voltage irregularities or other electrical defects may upset your computer, but it would not turn a hair (or a microchip) in the presence of a hallucinogenic drug like lysergic acid diethylamide (LSD). The human brain, on the contrary, goes literally berserk if exposed to even microgram quantities of such a psychotropic substance.

The clue, of course, lies in that very important gap, the synapse. The minute electrical impulse cannot jump across this gap, but must be transmitted to the second neuron or the other cell by the intermediate action of a chemical substance known as a *neurotransmitter*. As the electrical impulse reaches the nerve ending, it releases the transmitter substance which then diffuses across the synaptic gap or cleft and attaches itself to a specific receptor site on the other neuron or cell. This receptor is responsive only to that particular transmitter, and the result is to initiate a new electrical impulse which travels along the second axon, or to produce a specific physiological effect on a cell.

The nervous system, therefore, is dependent for its full efficacy on chemical as well as electrical happenings, and it is the involvement of chemical transmitters in this complex set-up which explains why drugs may have profound effects on neurological activity.

It could well be asked why the nervous system has complicated itself in this remarkable way. Electrical transmission has the obvious advantage of great speed and instant response, as shown by the rapidity with which we withdraw our hand from a hot stove. But electrical currents may run both ways along a wire or neuron. (There are not, I think, any biological semi-conductors.) The possibility of nerve impulses going *the wrong way* introduces an element of anarchy, and makes precise control of a complex system of interconnecting neurons rather tricky. Synaptic transmission, on the other hand, is a one-way street. The transmitter substance is stored only at the end of the axon and the appropriate receptor occurs only on the adjacent neuron (or on the cells of the tissue or organ acted upon by that nerve axon). This mechanism not only controls the direction of the nerve impulse, but allows the possibility of grading, modulating or even amplifying its intensity by varying the amount of transmitter formed and released.[1]

The disadvantage of chemical transmission, of course, is its comparative slowness. The transmitter substance has to diffuse, dissolved in tissue fluids, across the synaptic gap, causing a delay in transmission. This synaptic delay can actually be measured physiologically.

The concept of chemical transmission in the nervous system is quite a recent one, but it has had a stormy history.[2] It was first suggested around 1877 that specific chemicals might be liberated at nerve endings, especially those in the ANS. The idea lay dormant until 1907, when W.E. Dixon (1871–1931), Professor of Materia Medica and Pharmacology at King's College, London, noted that a toxin called muscarine, present in the mushroom *Amanita muscaria* (fly agaric), mimicked fairly closely the results of stimulating one of the two divisions of the ANS (the parasympathetic division). Dixon rashly speculated, and was laughed to scorn for his pains, that muscarine itself was the naturally occurring transmitter for parasympathetic activity. The idea of a mushroom poison acting in the human body was too much for most physiologists to swallow.

The opponents of the muscarine hypothesis were, in a way, perfectly right — muscarine does not occur in the body — but Dixon was soon to be partly vindicated by the epoch-making researches of Sir Henry Dale (1875–1968). Dale fully investigated the pharmacological actions of another chemical substance acetylcholine. This had been synthesized many years previously but set aside as a laboratory curiosity, and, of course, was isolated from ergot extracts by Dale (see Chap. 14, p. 100). He observed that acetylcholine imitated more accurately than muscarine the effects of stimulating the parasympathetic nerves. He also showed that acetylcholine had a very brief duration of action, and he postulated the existence in the body of an enzyme, which could split the compound and thereby abolish its physiological activity.

Definite proof that acetylcholine exists in the body and acts as a chemical transmitter in the parasympathetic division of the ANS was not forthcoming for some years after Dale's pioneer work. The main reasons were technical: the minute amounts involved biologically were impossible to detect chemically at that time. There was also, and interestingly, a fanatical opposition to the concept of chemical transmission on the part of a few reputable scientists, and this persisted well into the twentieth century even after much strong evidence to the contrary had eventually accumulated. The full picture of chemical transmission in both divisions of the ANS, the sympathetic and the parasympathetic, was not completed until as recently as the mid-1940s, and there are still some minor details to be filled in. Since many useful drugs act by imitating or blocking the ANS, the historical development of our understanding of its mechanisms will be described in the next few chapters (Chaps. 17–19). The ANS transmitters also play a role in the brain (along with many others unique to that organ), so these chapters can serve as an introduction to the later discussion of the psychotropic drugs and the principles of psychopharmacology (Chap. 20, p. 139 onwards).

For anatomical reasons, the ANS is easier to study experimentally than the central nervous system (CNS) would prove to be later on. The nerves and ganglia (collections of neurons) of the ANS, and the tissues and organs on which the system exerts its actions, are much more accessible to the physiologist and pharmacologist than the corresponding structures in the CNS. For this reason, the role of the neurotransmitters in the CNS proved much more difficult to establish experimentally, and the overall picture is still far from complete. However, the answers we are getting so far not only clarify the ways in which many of the psychotropic drugs act on the brain, but also help us to understand what happens during drug addiction, and can throw light on the causation of certain types of mental disorder.

17

The *True Muscarine* of Sir Henry Dale

> The night before Easter Sunday of [1920] I awoke ...
> and jotted down a few notes on a tiny scrap of thin
> paper. Then I fell asleep again. It occurred to me
> at six o'clock in the morning that during the night
> I had written down something most important, but I
> was unable to decipher the scrawl. The next night,
> at 3 o'clock, the idea returned. It was a design
> of an experiment to determine whether or not the
> hypothesis of chemical transmission that I had
> uttered 17 years ago was correct.
>
> Otto Loewi (1960)

As mentioned previously, the role of chemical transmission was first established in the autonomic nervous system (ANS) because it is much more accessible to experimental study. The development of our knowledge about the ANS will now be described in further detail, partly because many important drugs act on this system, and partly because the story will help us later to understand the far more complex situation in the central nervous system.

The ANS consists of widely distributed nerves, or nerve plexuses, which supply or innervate important organs and tissues such as the heart, lungs, blood vessels, salivary and other glands, and viscera. It is responsible for the moment-to-moment regulation of such functions as blood pressure, blood flow, heart rate, salivation, sweating, pupil size and many others.

The autonomic nerves have a rather complex origin from the brain stem (the bulb-like expansion above the spinal cord), and from the thoracic, lumbar and sacral regions of the spinal cord. They are conveniently divided into two categories: parasympathetic and sympathetic. The parasympathetic outflow arises in the brain stem, travelling with certain cranial motor nerves (e.g., the third or oculomotor nerve which controls some of the eye muscles), and also from the sacral region of the spinal cord. The sympathetic outflow runs from the thoracic and lumbar spinal cord.

All autonomic nerve pathways, at some point on their journey from the brain stem or spinal cord, form a synapse in a ganglion from which secondary neurons proceed to the organ or tissue on which they finally act. Autonomic ganglia are important for two reasons: they are often visible swellings or enlargements which can be readily identified and manipulated by the experimentalist, and certain drugs are now known to act at the synapse in the ganglion.

The parasympathetic system is concerned with conservation and restoration of energy rather than its expenditure. It slows the heart, decreases blood pressure, increases movement and secretion in the gastro-intestinal tract (thereby promoting digestion and assimilation), and empties the bladder and rectum. The sympathetic system tends to have (though not invariably) effects opposed to those of the parasympathetic. It prepares the organism for action by increasing the heart rate and blood pressure, shunting blood to the voluntary muscles, raising blood sugar and dilating the pupil of the eye. To give a simple illustration, one is in one's most parasympathetic state after eating a heavy meal and relaxing back in an armchair for a post-prandial nap. On the other hand, the need to run away from (or stay and fight) an escaped tiger would arouse the sympathetic system.

Many glands and organs in the body (but not all) have a double autonomic innervation, sympathetic and parasympathetic, and the effects of the two divisions are often in opposition. For example, the size of the pupil of the eye is determined by the balance between parasympathetic activity which constricts, and sympathetic activity which dilates, the pupil. This type of dual control is characteristic of many of the physiological systems of the body, and is admirably suited to the maintenance of internal stability (or homeostasis) and adjustments to external stimuli.

The ANS is not completely independent of other involuntary, or even voluntary, regulating systems in the body. Overall integration of the ANS occurs in an area of grey matter in the brain stem known as the hypothalamus. There are a number of nuclei in the hypothalamus; some, if stimulated electrically, produce a massive sympathetic discharge throughout the organism, and others produce parasympathetic discharge. The hypothalamus, together with some other areas of grey matter, form the so-called *limbic mid-brain circuit,* which regulates instinctual and emotional behaviour. In addition, the hypothalamus exerts a controlling function over the body's endocrine system via the pituitary gland, and has connections with an arousal system (the reticular activating system) and with higher centres in the forebrain, e.g., the prefrontal cortex.

These extensive hypothalamic interrelationships could explain how emotional factors might influence bodily functions, leading not only to transient autonomic and endocrine disturbances, but to a whole range of serious and long-lasting psychosomatic disorders.

The endocrine system is a purely humoral one, involving blood-borne hormones (or messengers) released from a gland and acting on distant organs or tissues. This method of control is obviously even more leisurely than synaptic transmission employing neurotransmitters, and certainly much slower than electrical transmission. These three different types of physiological control are, however, tightly integrated and coordinated at brain stem levels via the hypothalamus and pituitary.

This brings us back to the role of chemical transmission in the ANS. The brilliant researches of physiologists and pharmacologists which placed this concept on a sound footing were begun, and completed during the first half of the last century. The final conclusions were that acetylcholine is the chemical transmitter on the parasympathetic side, and at all ganglia in the autonomic system, and that noradrenaline (norepinephrine) is the corresponding agent at the sympathetic nerve endings (with a few minor exceptions). Transmission employing acetylcholine is usually referred to as cholinergic (*not* strangely enough, acetylcholinergic), and the nerves involved are called cholinergic neurons. Transmission with noradrenaline is said to be adrenergic, and we talk of adrenergic neurons. We also know now that acetylcholine is further utilized as the transmitter at the ends of motor nerves to voluntary muscles, at a site described as the neuromuscular junction. Release of acetylcholine at the neuromuscular junction (NMJ) causes the contraction of voluntary muscle fibres.

Acetylcholine is, therefore, a widespread and vital chemical in the body, and moreover, as we shall see later, it plays an additional role as a transmitter in some parts of the central nervous system. It was probably the earliest neurotransmitter to be elaborated during evolution, other transmitters being devised and made use of later as organisms became more complex.

One of the first steps in the unravelling of the acetylcholine story was taken in 1900 when Reid Hunt, at the Johns Hopkins School of Medicine in Baltimore, identified substances in extracts of the adrenal glands which caused a lowering of the blood pressure in test animals. One of these was choline, but the amount of choline present in the extracts was quite insufficient to account for the whole of the effect. There appeared to be another substance much more potent in this respect than choline itself. This other agent could not be isolated from the adrenal extracts at that time, but Reid Hunt spent some years looking for derivatives of choline with the necessary high potency. In 1906, he reported that acetylating choline produced a compound acetylcholine (known to chemists since 1867) which was 100,000 times more effective than choline in lowering blood pressure. Reid Hunt was greatly impressed by this fact, but assumed that acetylcholine was a poison or toxin formed under abnormal conditions or in disease rather than a substance with physiological functions.

Some years later, Sir Henry Dale also rediscovered acetylcholine, but this time in the fungus ergot which grows on and infects rye (see Chap. 14, p. 100). Dale not only demonstrated the presence of acetylcholine in ergot extracts, but showed that the substance produced two kinds of activity in animals. One group of actions was similar to those of muscarine, the toxin of *Amanita muscaria* (fly agaric), while the other group imitated the effects of nicotine, the toxic principle of tobacco leaf. Dale labelled these two kinds of activity *muscarinic* and *nicotinic*. Dale's investigations were, therefore, highly suggestive that it was acetylcholine which was the naturally occurring autonomic transmitter, or, as he said, the *true muscarine*. The expression *true muscarine* harks back, of course, to Dixon's earlier proposal that muscarine itself played this role in the body.

More direct evidence of the reality of chemical transmission in the ANS was eventually obtained several years later by the German pharmacologist Otto Loewi (1873–1961). Much of Loewi's research on neurotransmission was carried out at the University of Graz in Austria between 1909 and 1939. For his work on acetylcholine, he shared the Nobel Prize for Physiology with Sir Henry Dale in 1936. In an autobiographical sketch published in 1960, Loewi describes how he came to devise the ingenious and crucial experiment which proved that a chemical substance was actually liberated at the terminations of the parasympathetic nerves supplying the heart of a frog. Continuing the passage quoted at the head of this chapter, he wrote: "I got up immediately, went to the laboratory, and performed a simple experiment on a frog heart according to the nocturnal design."

Loewi removed the hearts from two frogs, the first with its parasympathetic nerve supply intact, and the second without (denervated). Both hearts were kept alive and beating in a special physiological solution, and the parasympathetic nerves of the first heart were stimulated electrically for a few minutes, causing a slowing of the beat. The solution surrounding this heart was then transferred to the second heart, which slowed exactly as if its missing parasympathetic nerves had been stimulated. This result proved unequivocally, according to Loewi, "that the parasympathetic nerves do not influence the heart directly, but liberate from their terminals specific chemical substances which, in their turn, cause the well-known modifications of the function of the heart characteristic of the stimulation of its nerves."

Loewi demonstrated this classic experiment at the 12th International Physiological Congress in Stockholm in 1926. With characteristic humour, he comments: "Like most experimenters, I had experienced time and again that experiments before a large audience often failed, although they never did in the rehearsals. Fortunately, I was able to demonstrate in Stockholm the experiment … 18 times on the same heart."

Loewi, like Dale, was unable to prove chemically that the substance liberated at the parasympathetic nerve endings was actually acetylcholine. However, the circumstantial evidence for it being so was now extremely strong.

The ways in which drugs can modify the actions of the acetylcholine involved in autonomic transmission, and some of the applications of these drugs in medical practice, will be discussed in the next chapter.

18

Fair Ladies and Ordeal Poisons

[T]he inhabitants of Eastern Siberia ... used *Amanita muscaria* recreationally for its cerebral stimulant effects ... The fungus was scarce in winter when, no doubt, the greatest need for it was felt, and the frugal devotees discovered that by drinking their own urine they could prolong the intoxication. Sometimes, in generous mood, the intoxicated person would offer his urine to others as a treat.

D.R. Laurence and P.N. Bennett,
Clinical Pharmacology (1980)

When, in 1914, Sir Henry Dale was comparing the actions of acetylcholine and muscarine, he noted that the effects of acetylcholine lasted for a shorter time than those of muscarine. He rightly guessed that this was because the physiological compound was rapidly broken down in the tissues, and he postulated an enzyme (acetylcholinesterase, or cholinesterase for short) which could split it into choline and acetic acid. This chemical change would effectively abolish the actions of acetylcholine, since choline had already been shown to have no more than one-hundred-thousandth of the pharmacological activity of its acetyl derivative. The later identification in tissues of just such an enzyme provided further circumstantial evidence that acetylcholine is one of the natural transmitters in the autonomic nervous system.

Opponents of the concept of chemical transmission in general had often asked what happened to a transmitter after its release, and why it did not continue indefinitely to stimulate the receptors. The answer to this is that there has to be some mechanism for removing the transmitter as soon as possible after it has completed its function. There are at least two physiological ways in which this can be done. First, a highly active enzyme can exist at or near the synapse which quickly destroys the transmitter so that its actions cease. A second mechanism, which operates in the sympathetic division of the ANS, is an active process of *re-uptake* of the transmitter into the nerve terminals whence it originated. In this way, the vital substance is *pumped back* to be stored for further release and action later on.

Another awkward question posed by opponents of chemical transmission was: if a transmitter is destroyed by an enzyme after release, how do the nerve endings get hold of further stores of it? There obviously have to be one or more enzymes for re-synthesizing the transmitter quite rapidly, and such enzymes have also been identified in the synaptic regions. In the case of acetylcholine, acetylcholine transferase is the specific enzyme present in the motor nerve terminals regenerating the transmitter, and storing it in little packets known as vesicles. This complex process actually involves many enzymes and requires metabolic energy. There is also a complex feedback mechanism which enhances acetylcholine production and release at times of increased muscle activity.

More indirect evidence for the existence of chemical transmission came from a study of drugs which could modify in some ways the actions of acetylcholine applied to neurons or tissues, or the results of stimulating parasympathetic nerves. Many of these drugs were of natural origin and had been used in traditional medical practice for hundreds of years. Some are still available today.

An early observation, made towards the end of the nineteenth century, was that when nicotine (the poisonous alkaloid of the tobacco leaf) was painted on an autonomic ganglion, synaptic transmission at the ganglion was first improved (facilitated) and later blocked (inhibited). Since acetylcholine is now known to be the transmitter in all autonomic ganglia (sympathetic and parasympathetic), it seems that nicotine can, initially at least, imitate the actions of acetylcholine at those sites. For this reason, Dale called these particular actions of acetylcholine nicotinic actions. Nicotine, therefore, turned out to be a useful tool for mapping the distribution in the body of autonomic ganglia, thereby helping physiologists to track the nerve pathways *to* the ganglia (pre-ganglionic fibers) and *away* from the ganglia (post-ganglionic fibres).

As long ago as 1869, Oswald Schmiedeberg noticed that the slowing effect of muscarine, and of direct electrical parasympathetic nerve stimulation, on the heart beat could be antagonized by the drug atropine. Atropine is one of the pharmacologically active alkaloids present in *Atropa belladonnna* (deadly nightshade) and other plants of the same family. Since muscarine is known to mimic the actions of acetylcholine at the parasympathetic post-ganglionic nerve endings, these actions were labelled muscarinic by Dale. There is a surprising specificity about the blocking actions of these plant drugs. Nicotine blocks transmission (eventually) at the ganglia, but not at the post-ganglionic nerve terminals. Atropine inhibits the latter, but does not affect ganglionic transmission. These facts have been, and continue to be, exploited for medical purposes.

The properties of deadly nightshade were known to doctors and professional poisoners in the Middle Ages. The Swedish botanist Carl von Linné (Linnaeus) named the plant *Atropa belladonna* from Atropos, one of the three Fates who cuts the thread of life, and from the Italian for fair lady, since it was used by women of fashion to dilate their pupils and make their eyes appear large and lustrous. This effect arises from an inhibition of the parasympathetic constrictor fibres to the pupil, causing an imbalance in favour of the dilator sympathetic innervation.

Atropine is still sometimes used to dilate the pupil in order to make examination of the back of the eye easier for the ophthalmologist, but it is commoner nowadays to prefer synthetic drugs like homatropine, cyclopentolate or tropicamide with a shorter duration of action. These drugs can also dry up salivary and other glandular secretions under the control of post-ganglionic nerves which release acetylcholine. A dry mouth is a characteristic result of giving drugs with atropine-like activity, and anaesthetists make use of this property when preparing a patient for surgical operation. Excessive production of saliva, and bronchial and other secretions during surgery can be inconvenient and possibly dangerous.

We have mentioned another site at which acetylcholine is the transmitter: the neuromuscular junction (NMJ) where it initiates voluntary muscle contraction. The blocking drugs here are different again. Some of the earliest poisons known to man were the herbal arrow poisons used in hunting animals by the Indians along the Amazon and Orinoco Rivers in South America. These poisons were generically described as curare, and samples turned up in Europe very soon after the discovery of the Americas, brought there by Sir Walter Raleigh among others. Claude Bernard, between 1850 and 1856, was one of the first to analyze carefully its mode of action. He showed, by a series of ingenious experiments, that curare acted, neither on the spinal cord, nor directly on the muscle, but at some point in between, e.g., the motor nerve itself. It was Bernard's pupil Vulpian (1826–87) who pinpointed the site of action as the neuromuscular synapse. Bernard and Vulpian did not realize, of course, the involvement of acetylcholine there.

Blocking transmission at the NMJ leads to paralysis of voluntary muscles. Curare, and the more recent synthetic drugs with this action, are useful, therefore, in capturing wild animals for zoos or in surgical operations to induce muscle relaxation for the benefit of the surgeon.

If doctors want, as they occasionally do, to promote or stimulate (not block) parasympathetic activity, it might be thought that acetylcholine itself, the natural transmitter, would be the ideal agent. However, it has grave disadvantages; its actions are too widespread and varied, and anyway last for only a short time owing to its rapid destruction by cholinesterase in the tissues. Certain natural drugs can imitate the actions of acetylcholine, especially at the terminations of the post-ganglionic parasympathetic fibres. Apart from the muscarine in *Amanita muscaria* (fly agaric), there is pilocarpine in an American shrub *Pilocarpus jaborandi* and arecoline in the betel nut *Areca catechu*. These agents have all been widely used in folk medicine, e.g., *Pilocarpus* to stimulate copious salivation, betel nut to expel intestinal worms, and betel nut and fly agaric to promote a pleasurable intoxication and stimulation of the CNS. Presumably these effects on the brain are also due to an action on acetylcholine receptors there, since similar effects are produced by injecting acetylcholine in cats. Moreover, these central responses are reduced or blocked by atropine.

The inebriating effects of fly agaric were popular among the prehistoric peoples of eastern Siberia, and later the Vikings used the mushroom to stimulate frenzy in battle. The betel that is chewed in the East (the Indian subcontinent and East India) is actually a mixture of betel nut, lime from shells and the leaves of a pepper plant (known as *supari* in India).[1] The mixture stimulates salivary glands and the CNS, but unfortunately stains the teeth black. The lime, which hydrolyzes the arecoline in betel to the CNS stimulant arecaidine, is also probably responsible for the development of oral cancer. For this reason, the Indian Ministry of Information now bans all advertisements for betel nut preparations.[2]

These age-old medicaments are no longer useful, and instead we have a number of synthetic substitutes, usually compounds of choline with some other acid besides acetic acid. A drug carbachol (carbamylcholine), for example, has the advantage of being resistant to cholinesterase so that its action is prolonged, and it has pronounced stimulant actions on the urinary bladder and the intestines. Such actions may be valuable after severe surgical operations when bowel and bladder function may be dangerously sluggish. All these drugs, both traditional and synthetic, are often known as cholinergic agents, and overdosage can obviously be conveniently treated by administering the blocking drug atropine.

There is, of course, another way to stimulate parasympathetic activity. Any drug which inhibits the action of the enzyme cholinesterase will prevent the destruction of tissue acetylcholine, and so enhance and prolong its activity. Such drugs are known as cholinesterase inhibitors. Since cholinesterase inhibitors will prevent acetylcholine destruction at all sites at which it is liberated, the actions of these drugs are widespread and potentially lethal. Early effects of poisoning with them are vomiting, abdominal pains, colic, diarrhoea, sweating, salivation and pupil constriction. Excess acetylcholine at the NMJ causes muscle twitching, weakness and eventual paralysis. Cholinesterase inhibitors, which are tertiary amines (e.g., physostigmine), can cross the blood-brain barrier because they are less strongly basic than the quaternary amine members of the group (e.g., neostigmine). So physostigmine and similar agents can also cause mental confusion, apprehension, restlessness, tremors and finally convulsions.

Again, plants with this enzyme-blocking activity have been known since time immemorial. The dried ripe seed of the climbing plant *Physostigma venenosum*, which grows on river banks in tropical West Africa, is known as the Calabar bean or ordeal bean. Its active alkaloid was isolated in 1864 and called physostigmine, or sometimes eserine (from an alternative name for the bean, Eseré nut). West African tribes used the Calabar bean as an ordeal poison in ritual trials for witchcraft. It is supposed that the legal diagnostic factor was the degree of salivation in the accused. The guilty person, his mouth desiccated by fear, produced less saliva than the innocent who experienced the full cholinergic effects of the physostigmine.

Today, synthetic cholinesterase inhibitors, e.g., pyridostigmine, neostigmine, and organophosphorus compounds, have several important medical applications. They will antagonize the actions of the neuromusclar blocking agents of the curare type, and so can be used by anaesthetists as antidotes to restore normal muscle function after an operation during which curare-like agents have been administered. Myasthenia gravis is a rare condition in which the sufferer has episodes of weakness and rapid tiring of voluntary muscles, especially those in the eye and jaw region. The disease is thought to be a so-called autoimmune disorder in which the body's immune system destroys its own cells, in this case the acetylcholine receptors at the neuromuscular junction. Not surprisingly, the symptoms are not unlike those of curare poisoning, and cholinesterase inhibitors will dramatically relieve the patient's distressing symptoms.

In acute glaucoma the pressure of the fluid in the eye (the aqueous humour) is raised above normal, leading inexorably to the loss of vision. The aqueous humour can be encouraged to drain away from the eye more rapidly, for anatomical reasons, when the pupil is constricted than when it is dilated. A cholinesterase inhibitor will constrict the pupil, promote increased drainage of the aqueous humour and, therefore, relieve the increased intra-ocular pressure. Atropine, on the other hand, will dilate the pupil and dangerously exacerbate an abnormally high intra-ocular pressure.

Powerful cholinesterase inhibitors, e.g., parathion, have been used as pesticides in agriculture (see Chap. 15, p. 105), as insects are very sensitive to excess levels of acetylcholine in the body. They have also been intensively investigated, unfortunately, as chemical warfare agents (the so-called nerve gases, e.g., sarin) by the military establishments of the world powers. Even pharmacology can be exploited for evil ends.

19

Fright, Flight or Fight

I was chiefly concerned, however, with the difficulty
created for Elliott's theory of adrenaline as the
sympathetic transmitter ... by the fact that noradrenaline
seemed to be much more accurately sympathomimetic.
Doubtless I ought to have seen that noradrenaline might
be the main transmitter — that Elliott's theory might
be right in principle but faulty only in the detail.

Sir Henry Dale (1953)

Noradrenaline is the principal transmitter released at the ends of
sympathetic nerves in the body. To establish this simple fact proved to be
much more troublesome for investigators than the corresponding problem
with acetylcholine and the parasympathetic system. The main reason
historically for this was the prior discovery of the very closely related
substance adrenaline, whose actions appeared to imitate with reasonable
faithfulness those of electrical stimulation of the sympathetic division of
the ANS.

If noradrenaline had happened to be identified first in tissues, then
probably it would have been given a biological name in its own right, e.g.,
sympathin. Adrenaline would later have become known as methyl-
sympathin, since the only difference between the two compounds is the
presence or absence of a methyl group (CH_3) on the nitrogen atom in the
molecule. However, adrenaline was detected first in 1894 in extracts from
two small glands called the adrenals which are found in close proximity to
the kidneys. The derivation of the chemical name is obvious. The
alternative name epinephrine, used in the US, Canada, Japan and Spain, is

merely a Greek translation (*epi* plus *nephros*) of the Latin (*ad* plus *renum*). When noradrenaline was identified later, it was distinguished from adrenaline by the prefix nor, which is an abbreviation of the German *N ohne Radikal* or nitrogen without a radical. This refers to the absence in noradrenaline of the methyl group on the nitrogen atom.

Epinephrine came to be used in the USA for the following reason. J.J. Abel (1857–1938), Professor of Pharmacology at Johns Hopkins Hospital, Baltimore, preferred *epi* and *nephros* at the suggestion of a Professor of Anatomy in Vienna, who quoted Molière's remark: "Parce qu'avec du grec on a toujours raison". Apart from the countries mentioned above, most of the rest of the world favours adrenaline (see Chap. 8, p. 62).

The discovery in 1894 of a substance present in adrenal extracts with an extraordinary potency in raising the blood pressure must have been one of the most dramatic in medical history. A physician practising in London, England, Dr. G. Oliver, was in the habit of using his family as experimental guinea pigs to investigate the actions of extracts of various glands and tissues. He had noticed that when he injected glycerol extracts of a calf adrenal gland under the skin of his young son, there was a marked narrowing of the radial artery at the wrist. Dr. Oliver gained access to a distinguished Professor of Physiology, Sir Edward Sharpey-Schafer, who was sceptical of these observations, but finally agreed, reluctantly, to test the adrenal extract on a dog which had been prepared for blood pressure recordings. Expecting no response at all and the consequent embarrassment of the humble practitioner, Sharpey-Schafer must have witnessed with amazement and incredulity the rise of the mercury in his pressure recording equipment to unprecedented heights.

The substance responsible for this action on the blood pressure was, of course, adrenaline, which came thereby to be accepted as a physiological agent of great importance. Its other actions were then fully studied, and the apparent correspondence between them and the effects of sympathetic nerve stimulation soon came to light. In 1907, Walter Dixon (1871–1931), the Cambridge pharmacologist, put adrenaline forward as the candidate for transmitter in the sympathetic nervous system.

Soon afterwards, Sir Henry Dale began to apply his acute mind to the problem of sympathetic transmission, and although he quickly realized that noradrenaline was a more accurate imitator of sympathetic activity than adrenaline, he never made the leap to the truth. The main reason, undoubtedly, was that noradrenaline was not recognized at that time to be a natural constituent of tissues, but was regarded as a laboratory artefact.

The amounts of noradrenaline in tissues are so small that science had to await the development of much more sensitive methods of analysis before direct chemical identification and measurement became possible.

Dale's interest in adrenaline was further stimulated by his work on ergot extracts. During putrefaction of these extracts, certain substances were formed which, like adrenaline, could raise the blood pressure of the test animals. These substances were described by Dale as sympatho-mimetic amines, since they also imitate more or less the results of sympathetic stimulation. However, none of these amines (e.g., tyramine) was a sufficiently accurate mimic to persuade Dale to champion it as a candidate for chemical transmitter. Ergot extracts also contain the alkaloid ergotoxine, and Dale found this to have the ability to block or inhibit some of the actions of adrenaline on tissues. Ergotoxine is one of the few examples of a naturally occurring inhibitor of the sympathetic, but in recent years a whole series of synthetic inhibitors have been discovered which have found wide application in medical practice.

The controversy over the true nature of the sympathetic transmitter continued well into the 1940s. As is often the case in science when a simple solution is being overlooked, the generally accepted, but erroneous, hypothesis becomes highly elaborated in desperate attempts to account for the experimental difficulties and discrepancies that arise. It was suggested, for example, that the released adrenaline combined with different tissue components at different sites in the sympathetic nervous system, and that it was the adrenaline-tissue component complex which produced the exact sympathetic actions. Even experimental results proved at times difficult to duplicate in different laboratories. This was eventually attributed to the presence in commercial samples of adrenaline (unknown to manufacturer and experimentalist alike) of variable amounts of noradrenaline as impurity.

By 1946 order had been restored, largely due to the efforts of the Swedish pharmacologist and physiologist U.S. von Euler. He and others established that noradrenaline definitely occurs in the body, and is, in fact, an intermediate on the biochemical pathway from the amino acid phenyl-alanine to adrenaline itself. In other words, there are tissue enzymes which convert phenylalanine to noradrenaline and can then add a methyl group to form adrenaline.

Although it is now clear that noradrenaline is the principal transmitter at sympathetic nerve endings, adrenaline has by no means been deprived of functional importance in the body. Adrenaline is released into the blood stream from the adrenal glands (actually from their central region known as the medulla which is a modified autonomic ganglion stimulated by acetylcholine), and acts essentially as a hormone to augment sympathetic activity in moments of great stress when fight or flight is called for. For this reason, adrenaline has certain special and powerful effects shown only to a minor degree by noradrenaline: increase of heart rate and output of blood from the heart; increased blood supply to the voluntary muscles; a stimulant action on the central nervous system, causing increased alertness and feelings of anxiety and tension; and certain effects on metabolism, e. g., release of glucose into the blood and increased consumption of oxygen by the tissues. Noradrenaline can be regarded as the transmitter for the localized regulation of sympathetic activity at ordinary times, whereas adrenaline is the hormonal booster released throughout the whole organism at times of crisis in order to clear the decks for appropriate and immediate action. The well-known remark that a stressful situation makes the 'adrenaline flow' is not, therefore, inapposite. (No one, even in the USA, talks of making the epinephrine flow!)

Since both adrenaline and noradrenaline play important physiological roles, it is sometimes convenient to refer to the compounds collectively as catecholamines, a name derived from the basic chemical structure which they have in common.

As with acetylcholine, there are tissue enzymes which can inactivate adrenaline and noradrenaline after release. In fact, there are two, operating at different sites, but neither is as potent as cholinesterase. There is also an economy mechanism for the re-uptake of noradrenaline into the nerve terminals from the synapses. There are some drugs which can inhibit one of these inactivating enzymes (monoamine oxidase), and others which can block the re-uptake mechanism. Both groups of drugs will obviously prolong and intensify sympathetic activity in the body.

The slower tissue breakdown of adrenaline and noradrenaline makes it possible to utilize these natural substances in medical treatment, though great care is required because of their potency. Adrenaline can be given parenterally in states of severe asthma, or in the treatment of allergic reactions and especially of anaphylactic shock. Intravenous injections of adrenaline can be very dangerous because of the effects on the heart, and would be resorted to only in dire emergency. Topical applications of adrenaline, used as a haemostatic to staunch bleeding, are safer. Noradrenaline was once used in therapeutics to raise an abnormally low blood pressure to normal, e.g., in shock syndrome and after extensive surgery, and was conveniently administered by intravenous infusion in very low concentrations. It has been replaced by newer, more specific, cathecholamines and similar sympathetic agents, e.g., dobutamine, phenylephrine, metaraminol and others.[1]

In general, however, the widespread actions of these physiological catecholamines make them rather unsuitable for medical application, and it is commoner now to utilize natural or synthetic substances which have more selective effects. For example, a synthetic catecholamine isopropylnoradrenaline (isoprenaline) is particularly effective in relaxing the bronchioles in asthmatic attacks.

Poisons from the plant and animal world which act as stimulants of sympathetic activity are, strangely enough, less common than those with parasympathetic effects. Perhaps the reason is that, although such toxins could certainly provide a defence against predators, it would be tactically unwise to excite your intended victim to vigorous self-protective activities in the period before his death throes set in!

One such substance is ephedrine, the active principle of the plant *Ephedra vulgaris* and known to Chinese medicine since about 3100 B.C. under the name of Ma Huang. It is said to have been tested and approved by the legendary Emperor Shen Nung, and according to the *Pen Tsao Kang Mu* (Chinese Pharmacopoeia) of 1596 A.D., the drug improves circulation, causes sweating, stops cough and reduces fever. Ephedrine, which has some similarities to adrenaline and noradrenaline chemically, was first isolated in 1885 by Nagayoshi Nagai, Professor of Chemistry at the University of Tokyo. Later, the properties of the drug were fully investigated by the American pharmacologists Ku Kuei-chan (born in Shanghai, but educated in the USA) and Carl F. Schmidt.[2]

Ephedrine has been used in the treatment of bronchial asthma, and occasionally in the eye to dilate the pupil in ophthalmological practice, but nowadays it has been largely displaced by the newer synthetic agents. Like adrenaline, it has powerful stimulant actions on the central nervous system, and this would lead one to suspect that it must act on adrenaline receptors in the brain. In other words, adrenaline is a natural transmitter there. Amphetamine is a synthetic compound which also imitates selectively the central stimulant actions of adrenaline, and is a popular drug of abuse for that reason.

There are also drugs which can be used to block sympathetic activity in much the same way that atropine or curare are employed to inhibit the actions of acetylcholine. The few natural ones are: ergotoxine (which is a mixture of three alkaloids) and ergotamine, found in ergot extracts; and yohimbine, an alkaloid from a West African tree which once had an undeserved reputation as an aphrodisiac.

Most sympathetic blockers used in medicine today are synthetic products of the pharmaceutical industry, and they have wide applications in many types of cardiovascular disease, in ophthalmology and for some endocrine disorders. The goal, which has been very successfully achieved, is to devise drugs which block selectively a particular sympathetic effect (e.g., bronchoconstriction, disorders of heart rhythm), so that therapeutic activity can be made more specific and unwanted side effects are reduced to a minimum.

20

The Microchemistry of the Brain

Many forms of insanity are unquestionably the external
manifestations of the effects on the brain substance of
poisons fermented within the body ... These poisons we
shall, I have no doubt, be able to isolate after we know
the normal chemistry to its uttermost detail. And then
will come in their turn the crowning discoveries ... the
discoveries of the antidotes to the poisons and to the
fermenting causes and processes which produce them.

J.L.W. Thudichum (1829–1901)

Scientists began to study the chemical composition of the brain and
nervous system during the second half of the nineteenth century. A pioneer
in this discipline of neurochemistry was J.L.W. Thudichum, a German
refugee who settled in England and did much of his work at St. Thomas's
Hospital in London.

Thudichum's approach was rather naive in the light of modern
knowledge. He investigated the brain as an analyst might look at a piece of
cheese, identifying only the major chemical components. He could not
know then that the most important constituents in nervous tissue are those
which trigger neurological functions, the neurotransmitters; and that these
transmitters are localized at synapses and act at incredibly low
concentrations. The limitations of Thudichum's understanding of brain
function blurred his otherwise remarkably prophetic comment made in
1884, and quoted above, on the possibility of finding a chemical cause for
mental disease such as schizophrenia.[1]

To regard mental disorder as being caused by "poisons fermented within the body" was obviously an echo of what was known at that time about the actions of drugs like morphine, alcohol and ether on brain function. Detailed accounts had recently been published on their pharmacology by, among others, Emil Kraepelin (1856–1926), Professor of Psychiatry in Heidelberg, and Arthur Heffter (1860–1925), Professor of Pharmacology at the University of Berlin. The latter had made a special study of the actions on the central nervous system (CNS) of the mescal buttons obtained from species of the Mexican cactus *Anhalonium*, which contains the hallucinogenic alkaloid mescaline.

It is not generally known that Sigmund Freud was interested during his early medical career in the central nervous effects of cocaine, and used the drug to cure a colleague of morphine addiction. Unfortunately, the colleague became a cocaine addict instead, the first example, perhaps, of Freudian transference! Although Freud in later years developed psychiatric views which discounted a chemical origin for mental disorder, he, unlike some of his followers, was always aware that eventually the psychoses in particular might turn out to have a chemical basis and would, therefore, be resistant to psychoanalysis.

A more sophisticated understanding of the CNS is beyond the grasp of the conventional analytical chemist. It requires the combined expertise of biochemist, neurophysiologist and neuropharmacologist, and it is only in recent years that real progress has been achieved. Even the very existence of chemical transmission in the brain failed to win general acceptance for many years, though such mechanisms in the autonomic nervous system (ANS) were fairly well established, as we have seen (Chaps. 17–19). The reasons for this are the infinitely greater difficulties faced by the investigator who tries to identify the central transmitters and to determine their functions.

It is not easy to study a particular region of the brain in isolation, because the whole organ is anatomically so compactly organized and its functions so tightly integrated. This is in marked contrast to the comparative simplicity of studying other isolated organs or tissues, e.g., heart, kidney or even an isolated autonomic ganglion. Furthermore, we still lack precise knowledge of the structure and functions of many areas in the brains of higher animals. This has led some neurophysiologists to use lower organisms as models, e.g., the octopus which has a fairly large but simple brain. Such work would, however, expose one to the criticism that the results might not be applicable to the complex brains of higher mammals.

These various problems drove pharmacologists at the beginning of the twentieth century to seek purely circumstantial evidence by studying the presence and distribution of possible transmitter substances in the brains of small animals such as rats or mice. One obvious approach was to look for compounds which were already known to have transmitter functions elsewhere, e.g., in the ANS; and, naturally, it was adrenaline, noradrenaline and acetylcholine that were first sought. Analytical methods of exquisite sensitivity had to be devised and perfected to measure these substances in brain tissue, because the levels were likely to be low. The reason for this is that chemical transmitters are not only released in minute amounts at the nerve endings, but there are, of course, enzymes present which destroy them rapidly after they have performed their function at the receptors.

In fact, chemical methods of analysis at that time were quite inadequate to measure accurately the low levels that occurred naturally, though some refinements, e.g., the conversion of the transmitters to fluorescent derivatives, at least made possible their detection in tissues. Until the development in the second half of the twentieth century of radioactive labelling, autoradiography, spectroscopy and positron emission tomography (PET), and the refinement of separative techniques such as chromatography and electrophoresis, progress in this field depended on biological forms of measurement (biological assay).

Biological methods were based on exploiting the very potent pharmacological actions of a substance. These actions, e.g., the shortening of an isolated piece of intestine, or the rise of blood pressure in an intact animal, were compared quantitatively with those produced by a standard concentration of the pure, known substance. In this way, the amount of substance in the unknown extract from tissues could be fairly accurately determined. Biological methods of assay had the advantage of high sensitivity, and, if performed with care, had remarkable specificity, i.e., you could be reasonably sure that you were measuring what you thought you were measuring. Also the use of antagonist drugs could increase one's confidence in the accuracy of the assay. They were, however, difficult to carry out and very time-consuming in practice, and became virtually obsolete when more sophisticated physico-chemical techniques were developed.

Nonetheless, they played an essential role in the dramatic advances in autonomic pharmacology that revealed the significance of adrenaline, noradrenaline and acetylcholine in general body control (see Chaps. 17–19).

This could, indeed, be regarded as the classical age of experimental pharmacology. Its last great triumph was probably the discovery of the enkephalins (p. 93) in the late 1960s and early 1970s by Hans Kosterlitz and his co-workers. US scientists were also seeking, using the up-to-date methods, to identify the natural transmitters that act on the brain's morphine receptors. They were chagrined (and sometimes angry) to be beaten at the post by a team in Aberdeen, "an inaccessible (physically as well as intellectually) outpost in the wilds of Northern Scotland".[2]

Kosterlitz's approach was truly in the classical tradition. His team utilized an *in vitro* system — the isolated smooth muscle of the mouse vas deferens whose contractions, evoked by electrical stimulation, are inhibited by morphine. The specificity of such an inhibition can be checked by reversing it with small doses of naloxone, a morphine antagonist. The next step was to extract vast numbers of pig brains, obtained from local slaughterhouses, and then attempt to show that purified extracts could inhibit electrically stimulated contractions of the isolated vas deferens preparation, and that this inhibition was reversible by naloxone.

However, the finding of a substance in brain tissue which had demonstrable pharmacological activity elsewhere in the body was not sufficient to establish its functional importance in the CNS. It was essential also to map its distribution in the various regions of the brain. If a possible transmitter occurs at more or less the same level of concentration in all parts of the brain, it may have been transported there by the blood stream, and so have no real physiological significance in the brain itself. If the substance is unevenly distributed, and especially if it is concentrated in functionally important grey areas like the hypothalamus or the reticular activating system, a genuine role as a transmitter becomes more likely. At the time of the Aberdeen work, Solomon H. Snyder's group at Johns Hopkins University were applying post-classical techniques to this problem.[3] They were looking directly for possible opium (opiate) receptors, using radioactively labelled drugs. After some failures, they chose tritium (H^3)-labelled naloxone which, being a powerful antagonist, would be expected to bind very strongly to opiate receptors. Then a series of opiate drugs was added to radioactive naloxone-treated extracts (initially of the intestine, but later of the brain) to see if any of them could displace some of the bound naloxone. They found that naloxone was released (detected by radioactive measurements), and that the amount released corresponded very closely to the known relative pharmacological activities of the opiates added. Further studies in animal brains treated with labelled naloxone confirmed the presence there of opiate receptors, and of marked differences in the numbers of receptors in different parts of the brain. However, even this kind of evidence is still essentially circumstantial.

More convincing evidence was provided by autoradiography, a more precise visualizing technique applicable to thin microscopic sections of the brain tissue. Snyder, et al. treated such sections with radioactively labelled diprenorphine (the most potent opiate ever synthesized, so presumably the most tightly bound to the receptors), and found that practically all of this compound was bound to opiate receptors and very little to other non-specific brain areas. They also detected opiate receptors in the spinal cord, an important discovery.

Slicing the brain is obviously unsuitable for detecting receptors in the human CNS. When diagnostic medicine developed a visualizing method known as positron emission tomography (PET), Snyder was able in later research to use this to study dopamine receptors in the brains of schizophrenic patients (see p. 162). Henry Wagner at Johns Hopkins labelled a neuroleptic drug spiroperidol with a radiocarbon isotope C^{11}. This emits positrons that can be detected by the PET scanner. Human subjects showed strong labelling of dopamine receptors in the corpus callosum, and some labelling in the limbic system — the parts of the brain associated with emotional response and behaviour.

Further supporting evidence, again rather circumstantial in nature, is provided if, in those areas, specific enzymes can be found which can synthesize, and also break down, the suspected transmitter chemical. Such findings would strongly suggest that the chemical in question is there for a definite physiological purpose, and has not, so to speak, arrived by accident in the blood stream. This is the situation, for example, with the parasympathetic transmitter acetylcholine. It occurs all over the brain, but is present in higher concentrations in some areas than others. Moreover, in the high level areas, the enzyme choline acetylase (which builds up acetylcholine) and cholinesterase (which breaks it down) are detectable. It is surely also significant that known antagonists of acetylcholine such as atropine, and known potentiators such as physostigmine, do have effects on the CNS. Certain events in the brain, too, can alter the levels of acetylcholine there, e.g., during general anaesthesia brain acetylcholine increases, and during epilepsy-like convulsions it tends to decrease. It is difficult to escape the conclusion from these, and many other pieces of evidence, that acetylcholine must be a central transmitter, but direct and unequivocal proof is still lacking except for certain special synapses in the motor cortex which control voluntary muscle activity.

A similar position has been reached with the catecholamines adrenaline and noradrenaline, and with another one called dopamine. Dopamine is the compound formed just before noradrenaline on the biochemical pathway from phenylalanine to adrenaline. All three catecholamines are unevenly distributed in the brain, but there are significant differences between the three. Noradrenaline levels are highest in the hypothalamus, reticular activating system and mid-brain; dopamine is also present in those regions, but is most abundant in an area known as the caudate nucleus where there is relatively little noradrenaline. The functions of the caudate nucleus and of the role of dopamine there will be discussed in greater detail in the next chapter.

However, pharmacologists have looked beyond the regular transmitters of the sympathetic and parasympathetic systems. In fact, practically every substance which can be biologically assayed in low concentrations by its effects on isolated tissues or organs has been sought in brain extracts. It is almost a matter of some embarrassment that many of these have been found there, and, furthermore, show uneven distribution. These substances must, therefore, be put on the shortlist of candidates for central transmitters, although they usually have no known function of this kind elsewhere in the body.

Altogether, the number of pharmacologically active substances which have to be seriously considered for a role of some kind in brain function is now well into double figures. Some of these are amines (e.g., serotonin, histamine, tyramine), some are amino acids (e.g., glycine, glutamic acid, taurine) or small peptides (e.g., enkephalins, growth hormone secreting factor). A small peptide is a compound containing a few (2–20 approximately) linked amino acids. In recent years, there has been a spate of research into these neuropeptides which has led to some exciting advances in our understanding of the chemical functioning of the CNS. Already a substantial number (60+ in 1989 according to Snyder) of neuropeptides have been found with activity, but it has been estimated that those represent only about 10% of the total number present in the brain. It is unlikely that all these substances are simple neurotransmitters, facilitating the transmission of nerve impulses across synapses. Many could be so-called neuroregulators, modulating the sensitivity of receptors to the actual transmitter; some may control the rate at which transmitters are produced or inactivated; others may directly inhibit synaptic transmission (i.e., act as neuroinhibitors). There may also exist more sophisticated types of receptors that have developed during the evolution of higher species.

The microchemistry of the brain is obviously immensely more complicated than Thudichum could ever imagine in 1884. Its full understanding is a task which will occupy neuropharmacologists and neurophysiologists for many decades to come. The jigsaw puzzle of the brain has many pieces and very few have so far been properly fitted together. Some pieces are still missing, and may indeed be almost impossible to find. It is, after all, not improbable that there are important CNS neurotransmitters and neuroregulators which are present in quantities too low for chemical measurement, even by present day techniques, and yet have no pharmacological activity on tissues outside the brain. The question is then: how can you ever detect such a substance?

The investigation of chemical transmission and regulation in the brain is rather like looking for a needle in a haystack when you do not know what a needle looks like or what it does!

21

Transmission Problems

I seem to have been only like a boy playing on
the sea-shore, and diverting myself in now and
then finding a smoother pebble or a prettier
shell than ordinary, whilst the great ocean of
truth lay all undiscovered before me.

Sir Isaac Newton (1642–1727)

Drugs can produce potent effects on the central nervous system (CNS)
because chemical transmission is involved in the function of brain neurons.
Drugs, which are essentially chemicals, may imitate the actions of the
natural transmitters, or interfere with those actions in a number of different
ways.

A complete understanding of the mechanisms of action of centrally
acting drugs will ultimately depend on a full knowledge of neurotransmission in all areas of the brain. Previous chapters have made it clear
that we are far from having the final picture at the present time, though
research workers are making rapid strides in the field. Even if we had all
this knowledge, further information would be necessary before we could
confidently predict the behavioural results of drug action. We would also
need to know much more about the neurophysiology of the brain, i.e., how
the various grey areas, and the neurons in them, are organized to carry out
the motor, sensory, emotional and behavioural functions of the organism.

We are still, like Sir Isaac Newton, merely playing with pebbles on the
sea-shore, and have barely begun to explore the great ocean of truth beyond
it. However, in a few cases, we can correlate to some extent the known
functions of certain brain areas, the transmitters which are most important

there, and the ways in which drugs can influence function through an action on those transmitters.

In the previous chapter we mentioned that the catecholamine dopamine is present in the highest concentrations in the caudate nucleus. The caudate nucleus is one of a number of grey areas known as the basal nuclei, which lie just below the cerebral cortex. The development of our knowledge of the functions of the basal nuclei has been aided by one of Nature's cruel experiments: the disease known as Parkinsonism or the shaking palsy, caused by damage to, or degeneration of, these nuclei. The main features of Parkinson's disease, which is not uncommon in old age, are involuntary movements and tremor, difficulty and delay in starting a movement, and a special type of muscle rigidity. Since nerve tracts descending from the higher motor cortex are responsible for the voluntary impulses initiating muscle movements, it would seem that the basal nuclei play a vital part in the finer control of these movements by an action on those tracts.

It has been known for some time that patients who die with Parkinson's disease show a low level of dopamine in post-mortem specimens of their caudate nuclei (about 80% of the normal). The activity of the enzyme dopa decarboxylase, which converts dopa (dihydroxyphenylalanine) to dopamine, is also lower there. These findings support the concept that the disease is caused by a localized dopamine deficiency. The further implication is that the basal nuclei contain *dopaminergic neurons*, i.e., neurons which utilize dopamine as their specific chemical transmitter. This is not the whole story, however. It seems that there are two balancing control systems in the basal nuclei. The dopaminergic system is one, but the other has acetylcholine as its neurotransmitter. In Parkinsonism, the lack of dopamine shifts the dominance to the cholinergic side, and this is responsible for the peculiar symptoms of the disease.

This view is supported by the fact that a drug called tremorine, which possesses strong cholinergic activity of the muscarinic type, can reach the brain and produce Parkinsonian-like tremors (hence its name). Also, in the days before the role of dopamine was revealed, one of the empirical treatments for Parkinsonism was the use of anticholinergic drugs like atropine or its synthetic analogues. These, by damping down the cholinergic side of the balance in the basal nuclei, allowed the deficient dopaminergic side to exert relatively more effect. In this way, normal function was more or less restored.

Recent therapy has been directed towards trying to restore the deficient dopamine levels in the basal nuclei to normal.[1] To give dopamine itself, however, is quite ineffective, as this weakly ionized basic substance will not cross the blood-brain barrier to the brain. Much ingenuity has gone into devising ways of providing extra dopamine, or extra dopaminergic activity, at the appropriate site in the brain, so that the symptoms of Parkinsonism can be relieved. One trick is to give the amino acid precursor of dopamine, dihydroxyphenylalanine (Dopa or levodopa). This compound, being more nearly neutral than dopamine and so less ionized in the blood, can cross to the brain to be converted in the basal nuclei by dopa decarboxylase to active dopamine itself. A snag in this treatment, which works extremely well in certain types of Parkinsonism, is that dopa decarboxylase is present in tissues other than the brain. Much dopamine, therefore, is formed in these tissues where it may have certain undesirable effects on the cardiovascular system (disorders of heart rhythm and swings of blood pressure). A clever way of solving this problem is to give, along with the levodopa, an inhibitor of the enzyme which will not penetrate the blood-brain barrier. Dopamine is then formed in the brain, where it is needed, and not in the other tissues. Another advantage of this combined therapy is that the dose of levodopa can be reduced, as it is not wasted in forming dopamine where it is not required.

There are other ways of increasing dopaminergic activity in the brain. Bromocriptine, a drug related to the ergot alkaloids, mimics the actions of dopamine, i.e., it has dopamine agonist activity. This agent can reach the basal nuclei after administration and function as a substitute for the absent or lowered dopamine. Unfortunately, the drug has the serious side effect of producing severe nausea and vomiting. Amantadine is a drug originally devised to cure viral infections, but it was found, surprisingly, to relieve the symptoms of Parkinsonism in a patient with influenza and treated with the anti-viral drug. It turned out to work by stimulating the release of extra dopamine from dopaminergic neurons in the brain, thus restoring the balance between acetylcholine and dopamine pathways.

Another way to restore the dopaminergic-cholinergic balance in the basal nuclei would be to give levodopa plus another drug to block the enzyme which breaks down dopamine, thus increasing the dopamine levels by a different strategy. Unfortunately, the enzyme concerned is monamine oxidase (MAO). If the destruction of dopamine is blocked, it will be converted instead to the next substance on the biochemical pathway, noradrenaline. Although this substance is also destroyed by MAO, the overall effect of giving MAO inhibitors with levodopa would be to increase somewhat the noradrenaline levels in the body. This could lead to a dangerous rise in the blood pressure (a hypertensive crisis).

In recent years, a novel surgical approach to the treatment of Parkinsonism has been tried, but is very controversial both scientifically and ethically. It involves the transplantation into the appropriate region of the diseased brain of dopamine-producing tissue from foetal brains.

Another centre of grey matter which has been extensively studied by the neurophysiologists is the reticular formation (RF). Its function has been shown to be related to sleep and arousal by experiments involving sectioning, or cutting across, the brain at various anatomical levels. Because of its functions, it is also called the reticular activating system (RAS).

Sectioning the brain has the effect of interrupting the nerve pathways which are descending towards the spinal cord (SC), and those which are ascending from the SC and those parts of the brain below the cut. If the brain of a cat is cut through the mid-brain *above* the RF, the animal goes into a coma and cannot be aroused. If, however, the plane of section is through the SC *below* the RF, the cat can show signs of being either awake or asleep. Obviously, the RAS is necessary to waken and arouse the animal by an action on the higher centres in the cerebral cortex. If the cat with its SC cut below the RF is sleeping, it can be aroused either by electrical stimulation from electrodes placed in the RF, or by an external auditory stimulus such as a clicking sound. Both these stimuli, electrical and auditory, produce detectable events in the appropriate areas of the animal's cortex.

These experiments indicate that the nerves from the ears go not only to the part of the cortex concerned with hearing, but also send branch nerves (collaterals) to the RF. The neurons of the RF then relay general arousal stimuli to the whole cortex which alerts the animal to attend to these sounds. Similar mechanisms occur with the other sensory systems of the body.

The existence in the brain of an arousal mechanism is familiar to all of us. A mother may sleep soundly through a noisy thunderstorm, but will wake immediately at the faintest whimper from her baby. The *limbic mid-brain system*, which is concerned with instinctual and emotional reactions, also has nervous connections with the RF, and it is not only the sounds, but the emotional feelings generated by the baby's crying, which are the stimuli for arousal.

The two groups of drugs, the sleep-inducing barbiturates and the phenothiazines used to treat severe mental disease, both influence the RF, but in interestingly different ways. The barbiturate, pentobarbitone, given to an experimental cat, will prevent arousal not only by electrical stimulation of the RF, but also by external clicking noises. However, in the latter case, electrical events can still be detected in the auditory cortex, showing that the direct auditory pathways are unaffected by the drug. This means that the pentobarbitone inhibits neuronal function in the RF itself, and perhaps also along the branch pathways from the auditory nerves to the RF. For this reason, pentobarbitone (and other barbiturates) produce a deep sleep from which arousal may be difficult, especially after large doses.

The phenothiazine, chlorpromazine (Thorazine), does not block the effects of direct electrical stimulation of the RF, which, therefore, still operates. Arousal by clicking sounds from outside is, however, definitely inhibited, although, as with pentobarbitone, electrical events can be detected in the auditory cortex. This implies that chlorpromazine has a selective action on the collateral (branch) pathways from the auditory nerves to the RF. It explains why chlorpromazine, though producing profound changes in the CNS, does not cause sleep or impair alertness and the capacity for arousal.

But what transmitters are involved in these various pathways related to the RF? This is a more difficult question to answer, but certain extraordinary properties of chlorpromazine allow us to speculate a little. When chlorpromazine is used to treat schizophrenia, excessive dosage may produce as a side effect a tremor and a stiffness of the muscles very similar to what we see in patients with Parkinsonism. This suggests that chlorpromazine is acting as an antagonist to dopamine in the basal nuclei, thus precipitating a drug-induced dopamine deficiency there.

We may speculate further. In many cases of schizophrenia, the patient is in a very anxious and agitated state of mind, and would appear to be over-aroused by uncontrollable and bizarre feelings generated within his limbic system. If we can assume that chlorpromazine blocks collateral impulses from the disordered limbic system to the RF, just as it blocks collaterals from the auditory pathways, this could explain the striking calming effect this drug has on severe schizophrenic psychosis.

The corollary to this hypothesis is that if chlorpromazine is regarded as a dopamine antagonist, then the limbic system or its branches to the RF must utilize dopamine as one of its essential neurotransmitters. From this point of view, schizophrenia could be regarded, at least in some of its manifestations, as a disorder triggered off by abnormally high dopamine levels in the limbic system, i.e., is a disease of dopamine overproduction.[2]

It goes without saying that this dopamine hypothesis of the cause of schizophrenia has not so far been firmly established, in spite of extensive investigations since the development of chlorpromazine in 1954. It is regarded as more probable today that any dopaminergic abnormalities which exist in schizophrenia will turn out to be secondary to other, more fundamental, disturbances in brain function or structure. The trouble is that chlorpromazine, like most drugs, has a multiplicity of actions. It antagonizes, not only dopamine, but some other possible central transmitters, e. g., adrenaline, and histamine. Jumping to premature conclusions because chlorpromazine has antidopamine activity is a very dangerous thing to do.

The fact that drugs have many different actions in the body is as much a bugbear to the basic research worker in pharmacology as it is to the physician who wishes to avoid toxic side effects in his medical practice.

22

Chemical Nirvana

> The passionate desire which consciously or
> unconsciously leads man to flee from the
> monotony of everyday life, to allow his soul
> to lead a purely internal life even if it be
> only for a few short moments, has made him
> instinctively discover strange substances.
>
> Louis Lewin (1924)

Aldous Huxley, in his book *The Doors of Perception* (1954), points[1] out
that mankind has used drugs since prehistoric times to obtain what he calls
"chemical vacations from intolerable selfhood". Of all these drugs, the
most fascinating from a psychological viewpoint, though the least useful
medically, are the ones which produce alterations in thinking, feeling and
mood, and create temporary states of mind rather similar to those we see in
the severe psychoses like schizophrenia.

Drugs of this kind are, therefore, often referred to as *psychotomimetic
agents*, but they have also been called *hallucinogens* from the visual
hallucinations which they can evoke. In 1957, the psychiatrist Humphrey
Osmond coined the term *psychedelics*, meaning mind-revealing agents;
and this has come into vogue among those who imagine that these
substances can somehow expand consciousness, and open the door to
states of mystical enlightenment and the perception of ultimate truths.

Surprisingly, certain natural products with these actions were studied
quite extensively in the last quarter of the nineteenth century, long before
Timothy Leary, the notorious guru of the *acid* cult of the 1960s, advocated
the widespread use of the synthetic hallucinogen lysergic acid

diethylamide (LSD). A pioneer in the field was the German Louis Lewin (1850–1929) who, after a broad education in classical and oriental languages, science and medicine, decided to specialize in pharmacology and toxicology.

Lewin possessed great literary gifts and wrote many books and articles of general interest on ancient medicines and poisons, e.g., on those mentioned in Homer's *Odyssey*. In an obituary by one of his pupils he was described as: "Pharmacologist, toxicologist, medical historian, keen scientist, brilliant teacher, profound scholar, fascinating writer, a man of noble character, lofty ideals and loyal to his race and faith". He could quote flawlessly, without hesitation, in many foreign languages (classical and modern), and marshal facts from all four corners of the world and all periods of history. One of his most influential books, published in German in 1924, was entitled *Phantastica: Narcotica and Stimulating Drugs, their Use and Abuse.*[2] This described in both scholarly and popular style the effects of depressant and stimulant drugs on the mind. He wrote, of course, at a time when little was known about the structure and function of the different parts of the brain, and well before the existence of chemical transmitters in that organ had been revealed. Nevertheless, his comments on the many drugs used and abused by man throughout the ages are perceptive, in spite of a certain moralistic flavour reminiscent of Victorian writing. (Of course, Victorian society was also a very hypocritical one. Writers like de Quincy, Sir Arthur Conan Doyle and William Wordsworth, among others, regularly took morphine and other addictive drugs. See also Chap. 31, p. 223 on opium addiction among inhabitants of the Fen District of East Anglia, England, in early Victorian times.)[3]

Lewin did some experimental work on the curious properties of the Mexican cactus mescal or peyote, which was named *Anhalonium Lewinii* after him. In 1888, he obtained some mescal buttons, the dried tops of the cactus, and was able to establish the presence in them of at least one alkaloid. The work was carried a stage further by Arthur Heffter (see p. 140), who isolated a series of pure alkaloids which included the active hallucinogen mescaline.

At noon on July 23, 1897, Heffter swallowed a fair dose of the combined alkaloids of mescal, and observed his reactions.[4] One hour later, he reported: "While reading, green and violet spots appear on the paper ... After shutting my eyes, visual images occur which are initially pale but gradually become more clearly defined and brighter ... I have predominantly images of kaleidoscopic figures, patterned carpets and cloth, luxurious articles of clothing and architectural scenes." He continues: "The capacity for visual images lasts in this experiment for an extraordinarily long time. Even on the following morning, coloured (green and violet) spots still appear when I shut my eyes." Other effects of the drug were, however, less pleasant. His notes record dilatation of the pupils, dizziness, very distressing nausea, loss of appreciation of time, impaired hearing and a feeling of tiredness in the limbs.

In commenting on the results of this personal experiment, he wrote with characteristic scientific caution: "It is very likely that we are dealing with an action on the central nervous system ... At the present moment, I would like to leave open the question of whether or not any of the mescal alkaloids have a therapeutic value. As far as mescaline is concerned, the answer is probably no." Heffter did note the opinion of some colleagues that mescal would become popular amongst cultured people as an intoxicating drug, but added: "I think that this is unlikely because the results which I obtained on myself show that the side effects are so pronounced that they considerably spoil the appreciation of the beautiful visual images."

Heffter underestimated, I fear, the compulsion that drives certain people to seek bizarre sensory excitements through drugs, in spite of unpleasant and even dangerous toxicities which are inseparable from their desired actions.

Mexico produces other *magic plants* with striking actions on the mind. The mushroom *Teonanàcatl* (*God's Flesh*) contains the psychotomimetic agent psilocybin, and the seeds of a bindweed called *Ololiuqui* are known to possess a number of derivatives of lysergic acid, with properties similar to those of LSD 25.

The quite accidental discovery of the first synthetic hallucinogen LSD 25 by Albert Hoffmann is a remarkable story.[5] Hoffmann, born in Switzerland in 1906, worked for many years in the research laboratories of Sandoz Ltd, in Basel. In 1936, he began to study the chemical structures of the ergot alkaloids. It was not until 1961 that Hoffmann succeeded in synthesizing one of the most important of these, ergotamine, which is widely used in the treatment of migraine. However, already in 1934, the common structural core of all the ergot alkaloids was known to be lysergic acid, and for many years afterwards Hoffmann prepared a series of derivatives of this compound. LSD 25 was first made in 1938, but nothing or little was done about investigating its actions at that time. In April 1943, LSD 25 was brought down off the shelf so that it could be further studied for possible clinical application. The actions looked for, of course, were ones similar to those produced by the ergot alkaloids already in medical use, i.e., contraction of the uterus after childbirth (ergometrine) and relief of migraine headaches (ergotamine). Alarming effects on the CNS were not anticipated.

One afternoon, while working with small quantities of LSD 25, Hoffmann was overcome by a peculiar restlessness associated with mild dizziness. He decided to go home on his bicycle. There, he lay down and sank into a kind of delirium "which was not unpleasant and which was characterized by extreme activity of the imagination ... There surged in upon me an uninterrupted stream of fantastic images of extraordinary vividness and accompanied by an intense kaleidoscope-like display of colours. The condition gradually passed off after about two hours."

Hoffmann realized that he must have accidentally ingested, or absorbed through the skin, small quantities of LSD 25 which still remains one of the most potent hallucinogens known. He decided, therefore, to swallow the drug intentionally, and he chose the dose, a quarter of a milligram, at which most of the commonly used ergot alkaloids exert a reasonable therapeutic effect. Hoffmann's reactions were spectacular. After about 40 minutes, he noticed slight dizziness, unrest, difficulty in concentrating, visual disturbances and a marked desire to laugh. Writing up his laboratory notes became difficult, and he asked his assistant to accompany him home by bicycle. Hoffmann's speech was now impaired, his field of vision swayed before him, and objects appeared distorted as if seen in a curved mirror. He had the feeling that he was glued to the ground and unable to move, but actually he was cycling quite fast.

Some of the most disturbing symptoms were: dizziness; the grotesque mask-like appearance of the faces of those around him; a metallic taste in the mouth; and a feeling of choking. Although Hoffmann experienced periods of confusion when he was shouting insanely or babbling incoherently, most of the time he was able to observe his condition with the neutral eye of an independent witness. After six hours, his condition improved and only the visual disturbances persisted. All objects were bathed in unpleasant, constantly changing, colours, the predominant being sickly green and blue. "A remarkable feature", he reported, "was the manner in which all acoustic perceptions (e.g., the noise of a passing car) were transformed into optical effects, every sound causing a corresponding coloured hallucination, constantly changing in shape and colour like pictures in a kaleidoscope."

This sober and balanced description of the various effects, pleasant and unpleasant, of a hallucinogenic agent is in marked contrast to the later overenthusiastic effusions of the high priests of the psychedelic movement like Timothy Leary and Humphrey Osmond in North America. One of them wrote: "The accidental discovery of LSD in 1943 may well be regarded by future generations as one of the turning points of Western Civilization." Osmond predicted that "psychedelics may have a potential impact on society equivalent to the Industrial Revolution." In 1954, the writer Gertrude Stein's companion Alice B. Toklas published a cookbook in which one of the delicacies was made from another widely abused drug with psychotomimetic properties, cannabis or hashish. "Haschich Fudge, which anyone can whip up on a rainy day," she gushes enthusiastically, "is the food of Paradise : Euphoria and brilliant storms of laughter, ecstatic reveries and extensions of one's personality on several simultaneous planes are to be complacently expected. Almost anything St. Theresa did, you can do better … "[6]

This equating of psychedelic with mystical experience is a frequent presumption of the devotees of these drugs. William Braden, a reporter of the *Chicago Sun-Times*, claimed in 1957 that "the fundamental thrust of psychedelic experience is religious, and its fundamental challenge is to the forms of organized religion." It is true, of course, that the use of hallucinogenic and intoxicating drugs has been widespread in the religious practices of primitive peoples. The Indians of the American Southwest have, for example, founded a religious movement, the Native American Church, which uses the cactus mescal in its ceremonies. However, the writer Frank Waters (1902–95), who lived among these Indians and knew them and their beliefs inside out, asserted that the mescal cult is of quite recent growth. "It follows," he said, "the deterioration of Indian culture as a substitute for their own valid religion which has broken down."[7] The use of such drugs would seem to be, therefore, an indication of the decline and disintegration of a culture rather than a sign of renewal and growth.

It is more likely that genuine and enduring religious insight requires the spontaneous interest and attention of a free and unpoisoned mind, and cannot be achieved by chemical assault and battery with potent pharmacological agents. This is not to deny that such drugs, by breaking down our internal mental barriers, may lead to occasional insights, rather on the principle of the well-known saying *in vino veritas* (in wine is truth). Psychiatrists have found these drugs capable of stimulating the release of material from the unconscious mind, and hence useful adjuncts to psychotherapy. This, in fact, is their only legitimate application to medical practice, but being potentially dangerous they have to be administered with care and responsibility. For this reason, psychiatrists are reluctant to employ them.

The other property of the psychotomimetic drugs, their capacity to produce states of mind resembling psychosis, has aroused more serious interest. The hope has been that, if their actions in precipitating psychotic symptoms can be understood in biochemical terms, we may thereby uncover some clues to the nature of the "fermenting causes of insanity" referred to by J.L.W. Thudichum (Chap. 20, p. 139). The possibility of schizophrenia being a disease of dopamine over-production has already been mentioned in the previous chapter. We shall now discuss these points further.

23

Molecules of Madness

[T]he regulation of our behaviour by complex interplay
of nervous and hormonal effects represents the perfection
of millions of years of evolutionary adaptation ... As a
pharmacologist, I have to reject the notion that by
administering this or that drug we can harmlessly
improve on Nature, to make us feel better or perform
better, to make us smarter or less anxious — and all that
without penalty.

Jack Fincher (1979)

Obviously, Dr. Fincher is no devotee of chemically induced nirvanas for
the normal brain. However, an organ which is so complex in its neuronal
and hormonal make-up could reasonably be expected to go wrong from
time to time. Psychosis is now generally thought to be a subtle form of
brain disease involving deficiency or excess of specific transmitters, the
production of abnormal transmitters with psychotomimetic activity, or
abnormalities of the receptor sites. Disorders of neurotransmission are the
modern equivalent of Thudichum's "poisons fermented within the body"
which he postulated as the cause of insanity (Chap. 20, p. 139).

The tricky problem is to localize and define the precise nature of the
biochemical defect in the various types of psychotic disease. It is in this
highly controversial and competitive field of research that scientific
reputations have been made almost overnight, and as quickly unmade as
new evidence forces investigators to eat their words or their publications.
Since spontaneous psychosis seems to be unknown in animals, or at any
rate is undetectable, and the living human brain is unsuitable for direct

experimentation, only circumstantial evidence can be expected and hypotheses will inevitably be rather speculative.

The likely biochemical abnormalities in psychosis have been inferred from three main lines of research: studies on the pharmacological mode of action and the chemical structures of the psychotomimetic drugs; studies on the mode of action and structures of drugs useful in the treatment of psychosis; and, a somewhat more direct approach, looking for abnormal chemical substances in the body fluids of psychotic patients.

The fact that chemical agents like LSD 25 can produce *model psychoses* in man could be regarded as a hint from Nature to help us elucidate what has gone wrong in the insane, but it has also tempted scientists to indulge in unwise and unfounded speculations. The organic chemist looks at the structure of these psychotomimetic compounds to see if he can pick out any grouping of atoms with a similarity to the structure of a known or possible neurotransmitter. It is then assumed that it is this part of the drug molecule which is imitating, or interfering in some way with, the actions of the normal transmitter in the brain. This kind of exercise has certainly led to a number of fruitful hypotheses, but also to many blind alleys.

Bufotenine (present in toad skin) and psilocybin (present in some Mexican mushrooms) and the synthetic LSD 25 all contain a chemical grouping known as the indole nucleus. This particular structure is also found in the pharmacologically highly active substance 5-hydroxy-tryptamine (5-HT for short). 5-HT is an amine produced by enzymic action from the essential aminoacid tryptophan. It is widely distributed in many plants, e.g., it occurs in high concentrations in bananas, pineapples and tomatoes, and in animal species from oysters to man. The compound was first isolated by Italian pharmacologists from the stomach and gut of certain molluscs and given the name enteramine. At about the same time, Irvine H. Page at the Rockefeller Institute for Medical Research in New York was studying a substance in blood which constricted blood vessels. He called it serotonin, and soon this was shown to be identical with enteramine.

Page later discovered that enteramine, serotonin or 5-HT is present in relatively large amounts in the brain, and others demonstrated that its distribution in that organ is uneven and its concentration highest in areas involved in central control of the autonomic nervous system (ANS). These surprising findings put 5-HT securely on the list of candidates for central neurotransmission, and led to considerable speculation about its functions in the brain.

In 1953, the distinguished English pharmacologist Sir Jack Gaddum (1900–65) found that many of the actions of 5-HT were blocked or antagonized by LSD 25, a property no doubt related to the indole nucleus which they have in common. Gaddum speculated, rather simplistically: "It is possible that the 5-HT in our brains plays an essential part in keeping us sane, and that the psychotomimetic effects of LSD 25 [as well as those of bufotenine and psilocybin] are due to its inhibitory action on the 5-HT in the brain."

This ingenious hypothesis received a fatal blow when it was discovered that a brominated derivative of LSD 25, known as bromolysergic acid diethylamide, was a more potent antagonist of 5-HT than LSD 25 itself, penetrated the brain well after administration, and yet showed no psychotomimetic effects whatsoever. Not only that, certain other hallucinogenic agents do not possess the indole nucleus at all, but are more closely related to one or the other of the catecholamines dopamine, noradrenaline and adrenaline. Mescaline, from the cactus mescal, is more like dopamine or noradrenaline in structure. This is also true of amphetamine, which can lead to the development of a schizophrenia-like state if taken in excessive dosage. Amphetamine was once freely prescribed to reduce fatigue and to treat obesity by suppressing appetite, but its abuse potential has led to its withdrawal in most countries. Its pharmacological actions are probably not direct, but due to its capacity to release the noradrenaline stores in nerve endings in the central nervous system.

Then there is the curious story of the pink adrenaline. It has been known for some time that old stocks of adrenaline solution can develop a pink discolouration, and if injected into patients may induce psychotic disturbances. The pink contaminant is formed by the oxidation of adrenaline, and has been identified chemically as adrenochrome. In the body, adrenochrome can be further converted to adrenolutin. Pure, uncontaminated adrenaline in the body is hardly converted at all to adrenochrome or adrenolutin, but is mainly metabolized by a different pathway.

In the 1950s, some psychiatrists working in Canada postulated that in schizophrenia the normal pathway of adrenaline metabolism was impaired, and an abnormal compound which they called Substance M was produced instead. Substance M was tentatively identified as adrenolutin, after it was shown that nine out of 14 normal subjects injected with pure adrenolutin exhibited some of the symptoms of schizophrenia. These psychiatrists claimed, in support of their hypothesis, that the blood of schizophrenics contained abnormally high levels of adrenochrome, but this could never be confirmed by other observers. They also, more convincingly perhaps, demonstrated that LSD 25 could increase the conversion of adrenaline to adrenolutin, and this might provide a plausible explanation for the psychotomimetic effects of LSD.

One difficulty with this kind of hypothesis is that the alterations in mood and perception induced by adrenolutin, though striking, are quite unlike those seen in classic schizophrenia. In fact, one of the main snags about drawing conclusions from the chemical structures of the psychotomimetic drugs in general is that there are important differences between the model psychosis and the real one. Retention of insight in the model is one such difference and another is that psychotomimetic drugs tend to produce visual hallucinations, whereas in schizophrenia auditory hallucinations are more common. However, amphetamine-induced psychosis is said by psychiatrists to be the least distinguishable from true schizophrenia.

Does the evidence provided by the therapeutic successes of the neuroleptic agents enable us to understand better the causes of true psychosis? Speculations along these lines have already been described in Chap. 21 (p. 151), in connection with the effectiveness of chlorpromazine (Thorazine) in controlling the symptoms of schizophrenia. The dopamine-inhibiting properties of chlorpromazine support the hypothesis that schizophrenia is a disease of dopamine overproduction within the limbic system of the brain. But, as was pointed out, chlorpromazine can also inhibit other neurotransmitters such as acetylcholine and the catecholamines adrenaline and noradrenaline. A specific dopamine connection, however, has been strengthened by some recent work of Solomon H. Snyder, Director of the Department of Neuroscience at the Johns Hopkins Medical School in Baltimore. Snyder and his collaborator Alan Horn have demonstrated that when one builds a molecular model of chlorpromazine in the so-called crystal configuration (the one it conforms to when displaying biological activity), the dopamine molecule can be exactly superimposed upon a major part of the chlorpromazine molecule. Since the spatial arrangement of the atoms in a molecule is related to its capacity to bind to receptor sites, this finding readily explains how chlorpromazine can combine with dopamine receptors in the brain and thereby prevent the actions of dopamine released from nerve endings.

This evidence was further strengthened by measuring the ease with which a number of related phenothiazines used in therapy (including chlorpromazine) could assume the configuration that displays the dopamine structure. It was found that the ability of the various drugs to do this correlated well with their relative potencies as anti-psychotic agents. Even more direct proof of dopamine involvement was obtained when it became possible to label specifically dopamine receptors in the brain with radioactively-labelled compounds, and to show that it really *was* these receptors that were being blocked by phenothiazines. In fact, the potencies of neuroleptic agents in blocking labelled dopamine receptors paralleled very closely their efficacy in treating schizophrenic patients.[1]

Another drug which has helped us to understand the cause of psychosis is reserpine, originally isolated in impure form from the roots of certain *Rauwolfia* species by the Indian pharmacologist Ram Nath Chopra back in 1933. Chopra writes in his book *Indigenous Drugs of India*: "The root of *Rauwolfia serpentina* has been much valued in India and the Malayan Peninsula from very ancient times as an antidote for the bites of poisonous reptiles and the stings of insects ... In the United Provinces and Bihar, the drug is sold as *pagal-ka-dawa* (insanity-specific), and its use is common among the practitioners of indigenous (Ayurvedic) medicine." Rauwolfia was revived in India in 1931 for the treatment of high blood pressure and schizophrenia. The active principle, reserpine, was rediscovered and purified in the West in 1952 by three Swiss scientists working in the laboratories of the drug firm Ciba, and was used therapeutically soon afterwards by the American psychiatrist Nathan Kline. Scientific studies revealed that reserpine binds strongly to dopamine and noradrenaline storage vesicles in the central and peripheral adrenergic neurones, and remains there for some time. This destroys the vesicles, and the nerve endings lose their ability to concentrate and store dopamine and noradrenaline. These neurotransmitters remain in the fluid surrounding the nerve endings (the cytoplasm) and are destroyed by cytoplasmic enzymes, e.g., monoamine oxidase. Similar effects seem to occur in serotoninergic neurones involving the neurotransmitter 5-HT. Clearly, reserpine, like chlorpromazine, has actions affecting more than one transmitter, but the important one is probably that against noradrenaline, and its overall effect is to deplete levels of that substance in adrenergic neurones.

Reserpine, though a herbal product, gives rise to side effects more serious than those of the synthetic chlorpromazine. It causes a weakening of the heart muscle (cardiomyopathy) which can make the subject a poor risk during surgical operation. Like chlorpromazine, reserpine can produce

Parkinsonian tremors, but, unlike chlorpromazine, it does not block the bile ducts in the liver leading to consequent jaundice. Moreover, reserpine has the strange and disconcerting ability to precipitate episodes of severe mental depression which may lead to suicide. For these reasons, the drug is little used today in medicine, except occasionally as a treatment for high blood pressure. It is the mood change that has aroused the interest of those studying the causes of mental disorder.

Mental depression is one symptom of a group of psychoses known as the affective disorders in which the patient shows extreme alterations of mood rather than the perceptual distortions of schizophrenia. No adequate reason can be found in the life events of the patient to explain this depression, which comes out of the blue. Sometimes the patient shows alternating moods of severe depression and manic excitement, the so-called manic-depressive psychosis (bipolar disorder). Actually, psychiatrists find it difficult to make a clear-cut differentiation between the various types of depressive and manic-depressive psychoses, but the action of reserpine would reasonably suggest that depression, at least, may be the result of noradrenaline deficiency in central adrenergic neurones.

If this is so, then one should be able to treat depression with drugs that can restore central adrenergic activity by increasing the levels of noradrenaline. In fact, the two groups of drugs that have proved most useful in treatment are the monoamine oxidase inhibitors and the tricyclic anti-depressants, both of which augment central noradrenaline, though by different mechanisms. The monoamine oxidase (MAO) inhibitors block the enzyme which breaks down the noradrenaline released at the neuronal synapses and the tricyclics, e.g., amitriptyline, prevent the re-uptake mechanism which returns released noradrenaline to its neuronal stores for further use.[2] To complete the line-up of evidence, manic states can be treated with salts of the metal lithium. The lithium ion is thought to promote the noradrenaline re-uptake mechanism, i.e., its acts in a sense opposite to the tricyclic anti-depressants.

We have, therefore, two plausible biochemical abnormalities in the brain to explain psychotic disorder: dopamine excess in schizophrenia, and decreased adrenergic activity in depression. Is it possible to obtain direct evidence for these hypotheses by studying dopamine and noradrenaline levels in the body tissues and fluids?

To study changes within the living brain itself, or even in the cerebrospinal fluid which bathes the brain, presents technical and ethical problems. Attention has been focused, therefore, on measuring the levels of transmitters or their metabolites in the blood and urine of psychotic patients. Results, however, have been disappointing. This is not surprising when one considers that neurotransmitters in general act at incredibly low concentrations, and so any changes in their brain levels in mental disease are likely to be minute. Also, it does not follow that changes in brain levels will necessarily be reflected in levels of these substances in the blood or urine. These considerations will apply equally to possible abnormal transmitters in the brain. Nevertheless, frequent reports appear of strange new substances in the body fluids of psychotics. Unfortunately, in most cases, these substances turn out to have a trivial origin quite unrelated to the disease, e.g., peculiarities in diet or drug intake. Strict controls are necessary in this kind of research, and many investigators have had their fingers burned by ignoring this simple precaution.

The inconclusiveness of these researches and the ambivalence of much of the evidence quoted earlier in this chapter raise the possibility that the fault in psychosis is an imbalance of several transmitters in the brain, rather than a simple deficiency or excess of any one of them. There may also be abnormal transmitters with psychotomimetic activity which have so far not been detected. A complete understanding of the nature of the biochemical abnormalities in mental disease still eludes us.

24

The Neuroleptic Revolution

> With the development of modern pharmacological
> techniques, psychiatrists turned to barbiturates for
> extracting truth from mental patients, and to pheno-
> thiazines for subduing them ... [M]ental patients need
> no longer be wrapped in strait-jackets but may be
> injected instead with drugs, which, if necessary, may
> be shot into them from "guns" ...
>
> Thomas S. Szasz, in *The Manufacture of Madness* (1970)

Drugs like LSD 25 can, as we have seen, produce symptoms reminiscent of mental disorder, and there are other drugs like chlorpromazine which can relieve such symptoms. Moreover, chlorpromazine is an effective antidote for those who have taken an overdose of LSD 25, or who are experiencing a *bad trip* on that drug.

The synthesis of the phenothiazine derivative chlorpromazine (Thorazine) by a French chemist in 1952 led to one of the outstanding therapeutic triumphs of our times, and created a revolution in the treatment of severe mental disease. By 1954, the drug was being used by psychiatrists in France, Britain and the USA, changing the whole atmosphere in the chronic wards of mental hospitals. Patients who had needed physical restraint or who would earlier have been subjected to empirical treatments of doubtful efficacy such as electroshock, or heroic brain operations such as frontal lobotomy, were miraculously improved on these drugs. In some cases, they were even able to leave hospital and rejoin the working community under supervision.

In the USA, the number of resident patients in state and local government mental hospitals, which had risen to a peak of 550,000 in 1955, began to decrease soon after the introduction of neuroleptic therapy. By 1978, the figures had fallen to 150,000, only about 27% of the 1955 peak. This policy of *deinstitutionalization* and closing of mental hospitals, however, has not been an unmixed blessing. Even on continued treatment, (which is difficult to ensure, anyway), many of these discharged patients fail to cope with life in the outside world and may come to join the armies of the homeless in our big cities. Moreover, the side effects of the anti-psychotic drugs are many and serious, and may require medically supervised alleviation. The therapeutic optimism, even euphoria, engendered by these new agents led to societal consequences that were not foreseen at the time.

The parent compound phenothiazine had been known to chemists since 1883, but it gathered dust on the laboratory shelf until 1934 when it was tried out, mainly in veterinary practice, as a de-worming agent, urinary antiseptic and insecticide. A derivative, promethazine, was synthesized in the 1930s and found to be a useful and long-acting antihistamine drug, and also to be effective against motion sickness.

Chlorpromazine was tested pharmacologically by Mme. S. Courvoisier and her associates in the laboratories of the Societé Rhône-Poulenc, a French drug firm. This compound not only showed weak antihistamine properties, but, in addition, a surprising range of other activities. In fact, the versatility of its pharmacology prompted the U.K. trade name Largactil (i.e., wide activity). Some of these activities are: inhibition of acetylcholine, adrenaline, noradrenaline and dopamine; anti-emetic (prevents vomiting produced by drugs); and anti-pyretic (lowers a raised body temperature). Chlorpromazine also potentiates or enhances the actions of a number of other drugs which depress the central nervous system, e.g., barbiturates, morphine, and general anaesthetics.

Soon after its synthesis, chlorpromazine was used successfully by the psychiatrists Jean Delay and Pierre Deniker for the treatment of mental patients. This shot in the dark was stimulated by laboratory findings that the drug reduced spontaneous activity in test animals, and in particular that it impaired conditioned (but not unconditioned) responses in rats. This meant that it did not affect direct response to external stimuli (as the barbiturates would), but only responses related to previous conditioning and therefore linked with learning and memory. This was clearly a very selective form of central nervous depression (cf. Chap. 21, p. 151).

Since then, many other phenothiazine derivatives have been

developed, and some other groups of drugs, e.g., the butyrophenones, have been found to possess therapeutic efficacy in the treatment of psychosis. Because they produced a marked degree of calming in psychotics, it was usual in the early days to refer to these drugs as *major tranquillizers*. The term *minor tranquillizer* was reserved for drugs of lower potency useful in the treatment of the neuroses. This caused some confusion, and nowadays it is preferable to call chlorpromazine and similar drugs *neuroleptic agents* or *neuroleptics* and to label the other drugs, e.g., diazepam (Valium), as *anxiolytic agents*. Before we can better understand the profound differences between these two types of tranquilliser, it is necessary to clarify a little what we mean by the terms neurosis and psychosis.

There is arguably a continuous range of mental disorder, with no sharp boundary between severe neurosis and mild psychosis, but an important diagnostic feature for psychiatrists is the question of insight. As a general rule, with the usual exceptions, a neurotic has insight into his condition, a psychotic has not. In neurosis, the subject reacts inadequately to certain stressful life situations and develops anxiety states, irrational feelings of panic, insomnia, depression or agitation, suicidal tendencies and so on. But he *knows* that his feelings are stupid, and no doubt tries to follow his friends' advice to *pull himself together*. The disorder, therefore, is essentially behavioural, and in mild form, e.g., the lexicographer Dr. Samuel Johnson's obsessional urge when walking along a street to lay his hand carefully on every post he passed, leads to no more than an amusing eccentricity of conduct. In more severe form, however, with panic states like agoraphobia (fear of open spaces) and risk of suicide, neurosis has to be regarded as a serious condition, and may benefit from drug treatment.

Psychosis, on the other hand, involves actual distortions of mental content, with delusions, auditory hallucinations and other bizarre sensations which seem frighteningly real to the sufferer. This suggests that in psychosis there are widespread abnormalities in brain function, especially in regions such as the hypothalamus and the reticular formation, and that these are related to defects in neurotransmission. In neurosis, the fault may be localized more to the limbic midbrain circuit which mediates emotional responses, and is a matter of misdirected, rather than disorganized, mental activity. This fits in with the fact that psychosis, but not neurosis, can be produced by clear-cut organic disease of the brain, e. g., in old people with atherosclerosis (hardening) of the brain arteries, and in patients with long-standing syphilis in whom the infecting organisms have damaged the CNS in a general way.

However, it is true that the spontaneous psychoses like schizophrenia do not have an obvious organic basis, since nothing abnormal in the brain can be unequivocally observed by the pathologist at post-mortem. This would not be surprising, of course, if the underlying fault here was merely one of deficient, over-abundant or abnormally active neurotransmitters or receptors. Also, the admission, even by psychiatrists themselves, that they cannot cure psychosis is consistent with this view, since no amount of talking and probing into one's early life is going to alter a biochemical defect. The effectiveness of the neuroleptic drugs further strengthens the case for a biochemical origin for psychosis (cf. Chap. 23, p. 162).

On the other hand, if neurosis is behavioural and related to faulty learning habits, it should be eminently curable by some kind of psychotherapy which can uncover those events in the patient's past responsible for the initiation of these bad habits. It is claimed, of course, that the minor tranquillizers or anxiolytic drugs are able to relieve neurosis. However, as we shall see in the next chapter, the anxiolytic drugs are not at all in the same league as the neuroleptics in their activity against possible neurotransmitters in the brain. Their therapeutic effect is probably little more than a sedative one, either with widespread activity like the old-fashioned barbiturates, or with more selective effects on the limbic system like the benzodiazepines (e.g., Valium) which are so generously prescribed by doctors today.

The greater potency of the neuroleptic agents implies, of course, that they are likely to possess considerable toxicity. Indeed, chlorpromazine has a daunting number of side effects, one of the most unpleasant being the so-called tardive dyskinesia. This tends to occur after two to five years treatment with the drug, and is a disorder manifesting as involuntary movements of the face, lips, jaws and tongue, and sometimes the limbs and trunk. The condition, highly distressing to the patient and his family, is difficult to treat. The intense toxicity of chlorpromazine has, needless to say, led to criticism of its widespread use in mental disorder, e.g., the psychiatrist Thomas Szasz has suggested that neuroleptics are merely a refined form of the straitjackets and other physical restraints of the past.[1]

To Szasz, there is no such entity as mental disease in the sense that there is, for example, liver disease, since the mind is not an organ. He regards mental disorder as societally determined, and nothing more than a deviation from behavioural norms. Neuroleptic drugs are, to him, society's latest way of punishing the victim (patient), and a convenient trick to avoid confrontation with the moral conflicts and social problems which (he supposes) lie at the roots of psychosis. Szasz does not, of course, deny the existence of organic brain disease.

Szasz's ideas are extreme, but they do serve to clarify our thinking about mental disorder and alert us to the possible abuses of neuroleptic therapy in our society. Richard Hughes and Robert Brewin, in their book *The Tranquilizing of America*,[2] quote many examples of the institutional misuse of these drugs in old people, the mentally retarded and juvenile delinquents. "The purpose," they say, "is not to relieve symptoms ... but rather to control behaviour through heavy sedation with unacceptably high dosage." Again, "The drugs are being used primarily, not for the medical therapy of the residents, but for the comfort of the staff." A special US Senate Committee reported that chlorpromazine (Thorazine), and thioridazine (Mellaril) account for more than 50% of all tranquillizer purchases for nursing home patients. It is said that among the elderly in institutions, 25% receive neuroleptics although only 15% suffer from actual psychotic symptoms. A recent comment from a geriatric physician at the UCLA School of Medicine summarizes the situation: "They're still using the wrong drugs, they're using them in high doses, and they're using them too frequently." We know, too, that these agents, and even harsher psychiatric treatments, were employed for the control (i.e., punishment) of dissidents in the former Soviet Union.

Szasz's views may have some validity for the neuroses, where there is probably no abnormality of brain function, but for the psychoses the evidence stacks up against him in recent years. Derangements of brain neurotransmission must be regarded as a subtle form of biochemical *brain disease*. Such brain disease could lead to a specific syndrome of sensory distortion and behavioural disturbance which would manifest itself as a definitive *mental disease*. Since brain and mind are intimately but mysteriously interrelated, there seems no theoretical reason why drugs should not be able to relieve at least the primary symptoms of psychosis by restoring biochemical normality to the brain. This point will be reconsidered in the next chapter.

The difficulty, as with all drug therapy, is to discover the selective agent which will normalize transmitter balance only at the exact site of abnormality. And, as we have repeatedly asserted, this kind of precise targeting of drug activity without any extraneous and unwanted effects is an ideal that is virtually unattainable.

25

The Age of Anxiety

I maintain that mental illness is a metaphorical
disease: that bodily illness stands in the same
relation to mental illness as a defective television
set stands to a bad television program …
[W]hen we call minds "sick" … we systematically
mistake and strategically misinterpret metaphor
for fact — and send for the doctor to "cure" the
"illness". It is as if a television viewer were
to send for a television repairman because he
dislikes the program he sees on the screen.

Thomas S. Szasz, in *The Myth of
Mental Illness* (revised edn., 1974)

One year after Thomas S. Szasz, Professor of Psychiatry at the State
University of New York in Syracuse, had published his controversial book
The Myth of Mental Illness,[1] the Commissioner of the New York State
Department of Mental Hygiene demanded he be dismissed immediately
from his university post. One can, I suppose, sympathize a little with the
perplexities of the rigid bureaucratic mind faced with the scandalous
existence of a professor of psychiatry who does not believe in mental
disease. That would be worse even than a professor of therapeutics who did
not believe in drug treatment!

Szasz's views, mentioned earlier, are that, although brain disease is an
undoubted fact, the concept of mental illness is no more than a misleading
metaphor, since the mind is not an organ like the liver or the heart. His
favourite analogy is to compare the brain to a television set, and the mind

to the programmes which it transmits. However, such an analogy, though striking and thought-provoking, can be pursued only so far, since the relationship between brain and mind is immensely more complex and mysterious than that between a TV set and its programmes. The brain, as an organ, is unique because it is aware of its own thought processes (or some of them, at any rate), and can to a certain extent modify them by its own apparent volition. Furthermore, it can respond to mental processes of other brain-minds, both directly and through the medium of books and other forms of indirect social influence. More debatable, but not necessarily implausible, is a possible influence of thought on the physical brain itself, especially in infancy and childhood when neuronal connections and networks are still being established.

It would be an extraordinary TV set indeed that could serve as a model for the brain-mind. It would have to be able to select its own programmes from a learned memory store, and, moreover, modify these programmes arbitrarily or under the influence of programmes it had seen on other sets. Its programmes might actually be able to alter the electronic circuitry of the set itself.

Brain without an active mind can be seen on the post-mortem slab, and mind without brain leads us into the realm of metaphysics. But surely we must accept that, in life, mind and brain can intimately interact with one another, and that both are possibly facets of some greater unity which cannot be grasped intellectually by one component of that unity, our mind.

In view of this, it is not surprising that the medical profession has always found great difficulty in deciding whether certain *mental* disorders are *genuine* or *put on* by the patient to arouse sympathy and attention. The *genuine* disorders, which can be related to a definite neurological defect or abnormality, are described as *organic*. Those disorders for which no physical cause can be detected are labelled *functional*, the implication being that the patient is malingering or (more charitably) is disturbed psychologically by stress or anxiety.

Doctors who can find no organic causes for a patient's complaints have always been rather too inclined to dismiss his or her (especially her!) symptoms as functional. In the past, for example, patients with myasthenia gravis or multiple sclerosis were dismissed as little better than malingerers, though today we know that there are real neurological processes underlying these diseases. With obvious organic disease of the brain, e.g., in neurosyphilis or after severe strokes, there is usually no problem of diagnosis, and the disorder is actually, or at least potentially, treatable by a member of the medical profession.

The difficulty arises with the psychoses in which no obvious pathological abnormality of, or damage to, the brain can usually be detected. Yet, as explained in the previous chapters, there is evidence that there may be some subtle derangement of neurotransmission in these conditions. If so, then psychosis could be explained, at least in part, in physiological terms and regarded, *pace* Szasz, as an organic disease of the brain. Moreover, the existence of such a biochemical defect opens the way to the possibility of medical treatment of some kind and especially drug therapy aimed at normalizing the disorder of neurotransmitter balance in the brain.

Granted all this, Szasz still has a valid point and his views deserve serious consideration. Even though psychosis is turning out to be biochemically determined, the symptoms of the disease are bound to be strongly influenced by societal and cultural factors. Perceptual abnormalities may distort the behavioural programmes of the mind and since these programmes have their origin in society, the reaction of the psychotic to his symptoms is inevitably coloured by the basic assumptions of the society in which he lives. To hear supernatural voices and to obey their commands must have been less disturbing to schizophrenics in the theocratic Middle Ages than it is in today's secular society. Much of the anxiety, the fear and the panic felt by the psychotic is probably a functional reaction to the primary symptoms of the disease. Obviously, these secondary symptoms are not in themselves curable by any kind of medical treatment, though drugs may produce some palliative effect by damping down neurological pathways in the brain (acting as a sort of pharmacological straight-jacket, in fact!).

To complicate the situation even further, these secondary functional symptoms, if persistent, can lead to tertiary changes in endocrine and autonomic mechanisms by effects *via* the limbic system and the hypothalamus. This implies the development of psychosomatic symptoms, the organic aspects of which *would* be capable of some degree of alleviation by drug therapy.

Neurosis, which is almost by definition purely functional and unrelated to any physiological or biochemical abnormality, is quite another matter. Here, Szasz's views surely come into their own, and simple neurosis cannot be regarded as a disease in the strict sense. Again, however, we must be aware of the possibility of secondary somatic changes in the endocrine and autonomic function caused by long-term neurotic tensions. In neurosis, therefore, drug treatment can be little more than a soporific or tranquillizer for the mind of the sufferer, so that he becomes less disturbed by the purely psychological and sociological stresses and strains underlying his condition, though drugs could perhaps help alleviate any associated psychosomatic symptoms. In view of this, one might well ask why the medical profession is called in to treat neurosis at all. Why not the priest, the social worker or even the psychoanalyst?

According to Szasz, the problem of how to deal with the socially and psychologically maladjusted throughout history has always been resolved in terms of the ruling ideologies of the times. In the European Middle Ages, when theological issues were predominant, misfits were often labelled witches or heretics, and burned at the stake if they did not recant. Since then, Western society has become increasingly secularized, and increasingly permeated by the values of natural science and scientific medicine. There has been in modern times, therefore, a tendency to medicalize the problems of the maladjusted ("he is a sick person!").

During the enormous growth of medical science in the second half of the nineteenth century, attempts were made by such outstanding figures as Jean Martin Charcot (1825–93) to classify in medical terms the various neurological and psychiatric syndromes seen in the overcrowded mental institutions of the time, e.g., the Salpêtrière in Paris. Out of these endeavours came the specializations of the twentieth century: the neurologist for obvious organic disease of the central nervous system, and the psychiatrist for disorders that were regarded, rightly or wrongly, as purely functional. Sigmund Freud, for example, studied with Charcot, and developed many of his psychoanalytic concepts from his observations of cases of hysteria under Charcot's care. Psychoanalysis, however, because of its unorthodox therapies, has always hovered on the fringe of established medicine and made forays into sociology, philosophy and religion. For these reasons, the psychoanalyst has tended to take over, especially in countries like the USA, the role of the priest and father-confessor to his patients.

But even the psychiatrist likes to believe that he is being scientific and medical, and that in treating neurosis he is treating a real sickness. Neurotic syndromes, therefore, have to be given pretentious diagnostic labels. Szasz, in a 1991 article "Diagnoses are not Diseases"[2] in the medical journal *Lancet* makes easy fun of this. The American Psychiatric Association publishes from time to time a *Diagnostic and Statistical*

Manual of Mental Disorders. The 1990 Edition (DSM-III) distinguished itself by removing homosexuality from its list of mental disorders, but still includes such monstrosities as "Body Dysmorphic Disorder" (a preoccupation with some imagined defect in appearance in a normal-appearing person). It also threatened that in DSM-IV (the 1994 Edition) premenstrual syndrome (PMS) would feature as "Late Luteal Phase Dysphoric Disorder". Better judgement must have prevailed, and in the 2000 Revision it appears as "Premenstrual Dysphoric Disorder".[3]

However, full psychoanalytic treatment is time-consuming and fortunately most of us cannot afford it. Consequently, the average neurotic today is likely to gravitate with his complaints to the ordinary medical practitioner. What can such a doctor do for problems that are not fundamentally medical in nature?

Drugs, of course, are the instant form of treatment, taking no longer than the time to write a prescription. That they are so lavishly administered is not, therefore, surprising, especially when we consider the magnitude of the challenge to the profession. Surveys in the USA and Britain have shown that between one quarter and one third of all adults have significant symptoms of psychological disturbance, admitting to nervousness, depression, irritability or sleeplessness. Patients with psychiatric complaints account for about 25% of all consultations with a medical practitioner, and of these only about 5% are eventually diagnosed as psychotics. The rest presumably suffer from some kind of neurosis. What Garth Wood, the author of *The Myth of Neurosis* (1984), scathingly calls the *psychotherapy industry* cost the USA about 3% of the total 1987 expenditure on health care.[4]

In a representative sample of 40,000 people studied in Britain in 1977, psychotropic (mood-altering) drugs were being prescribed to 10% of males and 21% of females. Of women aged 45–59, 33% received a psychotropic drug, and 11% were given an anti-depressant. All these drugs tend to have hypnotic (sleep-inducing), anti-epileptic or muscle relaxing activity, and cover a range from the bromides of Victorian times to the latest benzodiazepine from the drug firms. Their effect is essentially to blunt emotional response by numbing the brain and producing a degree of drowsiness and apathy. In the past, they would have been called sedatives, but are now more pretentiously described as minor tranquillizers or anxiolytic agents. Since insomnia and muscular tension are often secondary symptoms of neurosis, these hypnotics and muscle relaxants will incidentally relieve those symptoms to the undoubted benefit of the patient.

Many psychiatrists, needless to say, disapprove of any drug treatment for neurosis, believing that the condition is best not tranquillized, but accepted and discussed as a pointer to hidden conflicts which must be revealed and talked over for final resolution and cure. The ordinary practitioner, however, is in no position to deny these pharmacological crutches to his patients to tide them over periods of severe anxiety, and it would perhaps be cruel to withhold them.

Unfortunately, but not unexpectedly, these drugs have side effects, often serious ones. Bromides (usually a mixture of sodium and potassium bromides) were introduced in 1857, and administered (according to a *Handbook of Therapeutics* published in 1897) for "night screaming in children, townswomen who are going out of their minds … nymphomania and undue indulgence in bed". Bromides are exceedingly toxic, and have the disadvantage of cumulating in the body over a period of time even if given in very low doses (like the metal lead).

Bromides became obsolete as soon as the far superior barbiturates were synthesized in 1903, but these in turn were superseded by the benzodiazepines in the 1950s. Since these synthetic drugs are also useful as hypnotics, they will be discussed in more detail in the next two chapters on the pharmacology of sleep.

26

A Good Night's Rest

> At a very rough reckoning about one night's
> sleep in every ten in this country [Britain]
> is hypnotic induced ... People seem to want to
> turn consciousness on and off like a tap ...
>
> Sir Derrick Dunlop (1970)

Sir Derrick, formerly Professor of Therapeutics at the University of Edinburgh, Scotland, continued: "While it is time-consuming to take a careful clinical history, to conduct a full clinical examination and to give wise advice, it takes only a moment to write a prescription and this does please and often satisfies the patient ... We do not always draw a clear distinction between the patient's *wants* and what we think are his *needs*, and it is regrettable how much we accede to the patient's demands in order to placate him and to save ourselves time and trouble."

There is little evidence that these sensible views have been taken to heart by the majority of the medical profession. Some figures, from the *British Medical Journal* (1988) for the use of the benzodiazepine group of hypnotics have already been quoted in Chap. 3, p. 26. It is among older people, those over 65, that misuse of these drugs is particularly widespread. The 1988 UK survey reported in the *British Medical Journal*[1] found that 16% in this age group took hypnotics (mainly benzodiazepines), and of these 75% had been on them for one year or more and 25% for ten years or more. Some estimates suggest that 40 billion doses of benzodiazepines are ingested daily throughout the world. These drugs, of course, are not only used as hypnotics, but also to relieve neurotic anxiety (see p. 178). These two actions, the hypnotic and the anxiolytic, are probably based on somewhat different pharmacological mechanisms, and the possibility exists of eventually finding drugs with exclusively one action or the other.

Sleep is an inescapable need in man and the higher mammals, but its purpose is still far from clear. The average healthy adult sleeps about seven to eight hours a night, with occasional brief periods of dozing (*microsleeps*) during the day, but there are wide individual variations. Napoleon Bonaparte is said to have slept only two to three hours per night, and British ex-Prime Minister Margaret Thatcher flourished on four hours. Albert Einstein, on the other hand, liked a lot of sleep. This implies that insomnia and feeling tired are highly subjective symptoms and must not be taken at face value. Feeling tired can be due to other causes than lack of sleep, e.g., anaemia, and complaints of not sleeping well may only reflect the subject's opinion that he sleeps fewer hours than he thinks he ought to. Not only that, insomniacs typically underestimate the hours they sleep, or, rather, overestimate the time they stay awake tossing from side to side.

Insomnia in otherwise healthy people can show three rather obvious patterns. The subject may take a long time to fall asleep, but after that he sleeps well; he may wake up frequently and for long periods during the night; or he may wake up too early in the morning and be unable to get to sleep again. Whether any of these matters in the slightest degree is debatable, and there is everything to be said against resorting to drugs to restore supposed *normality* in these usually harmless forms of insomnia. Sleep requirements appear to decrease with increasing age, and nocturnal awakenings occur more often, but again this is probably of no importance and hypnotic drugs are not indicated. To recommend in these cases a small snack, a hot drink or even a mild alcoholic night-cap before retiring to bed is good advice, and very much less harmful in the long run.

Nevertheless, according to Wallace B. Mendelson (1987),[2] about 35% of the US population complain of difficulty in getting to sleep and maintaining it, although only half of them regard it as a major problem. Of those seeing a doctor, 4.3% get a prescription for a hypnotic each year, and of these roughly three-quarters take the drug for less than two weeks and 11% use it nightly for up to a year.

Insomnia with a clear-cut cause is another matter. Temporary sleeplessness due to the psychological trauma of, say, a bereavement, mental stress from overwork or being in the unfamiliar environment of a hospital ward may benefit from short courses of a hypnotic drug in order to restore normal sleeping habits. About 80% of patients with acute psychosis suffer from insomnia, and the complaint is common in neurotic states like anxiety and depression. These patients do not need hypnotics but specific treatments for their conditions, e.g., neuroleptic or anti-depressant drugs, or even psychoanalysis. It may be possible to relate insomnia to imbibing too many caffeine-containing drinks, and cutting out tea, coffee, Coca Cola, etc, late in the day may be perfectly adequate treatment in these cases. Insomnia caused primarily by severe pain cannot be relieved by hypnotics alone, but requires potent analgesics.

The important point is that a good practitioner should try to prevent his patients becoming unduly reliant on hypnotic and tranquillizing drugs because of the dangers of dependence. He must not evade the fact that drugs merely help his patients to avoid their real problems, and, being drugs, they have their inevitable side effects. To go into this further, we must first outline our present knowledge of the nature and purpose of sleep.

The normal patterns of sleep and wakefulness involve a cyclic alternation between several, rather than just two, dissimilar states of the brain. This has been revealed using an encephalograph in which electrical activity in the brain is picked up from electrodes placed at certain points on the scalp. The recordings obtained, known as electroencephalograms (EEGs), are exceedingly difficult to interpret, but have been used to detect brain tumours and to locate epileptic foci and other brain abnormalities.

EEG recordings differ according to whether the subject is awake or asleep. In sleep, the electrical tracings show certain regular features characterized imaginatively as theta waves, delta waves, spikes, spindles and K complexes. When the subject is awakened by an external stimulus, these disappear and the record is said to be *desynchronized*. The waking EEG does show irregular alpha and beta waves, but there are no longer obvious and recurrent patterns of activity.

A night's sleep can be divided into four definite stages of increasing depth. Stage 1 is the well-known drowsy state preceding the onset of actual sleep, and usually lasts only a few minutes. The alpha waves of the waking state are considerably reduced, and slower theta waves appear. In stage 2, theta waves increase, spindles and K complexes occur, and in stages 3 and 4 sleep becomes progressively deeper with the appearance of slow delta waves. These four stages are known collectively as *orthodox sleep* or non-rapid eye movement sleep (NREM). There is, however, another very interesting type of sleep which interrupts the course of NREM sleep several times during the night.

This is the so-called *Rapid Eye Movement Sleep* (REM or paradoxical sleep), and the first episode usually appears in the normal young adult after 70–120 minutes (average: 90 minutes) of NREM sleep. There is a lightening of sleep, and the EEG once more resembles that shown in stage 1 with no spindles or K complexes. Very characteristically, there are rapid movements of the eyeballs and the subject may experience dreams. Episodes of REM sleep occur roughly every 90 minutes during the night, i.e., there are normally about four to five cycles of NREM-REM sleep, but there is a tendency for the REM periods to increase and for stage 4 slow wave sleep to decrease in length towards the morning. In other words, one's soundest and most dreamless sleep occurs earlier in the night. Both REM and stage 4 sleep are highest in infancy and childhood, level off in adult life and decline in old age. Typically, a young adult's nightly sleep comprises 5% stage 1, 50% stage 2, 10% stage 3, 10% stage 4 and 25% REM.

What makes us fall asleep, and what wakes us up and keeps us awake, are questions which bring us once again to a consideration of neurotransmitter function in the brain. It is a matter of experience that we (and the higher mammals) require interest and stimulation to maintain our alertness, and that boredom, a dull lecture or an unexciting environment soon lead to yawning and an irresistible desire to doze. We have already explained (Chap. 21, p. 147) that active stimulation and arousal is a function of the reticular activating system (RAS). It is significant, therefore, that EEG desynchronization in animals can be produced by direct electrical stimulation of the RAS. Also, drugs like the barbiturates and alcohol can definitely depress the RAS, thereby causing a deep, unnatural sleep from which arousal is difficult. The transmitter involved in the neurological pathways of the RAS is probably one of the catecholamines, e.g., dopamine or noradrenaline.

All this might suggest that sleep is a purely passive process which supervenes automatically when stimuli from the RAS fall below a certain level of intensity. This view became suspect after it was shown that direct electrical stimulation of various areas of the brain could induce sleep,[3] and quite untenable when the sleep process was demonstrated to be a phenomenon of great complexity involving REM and various stages of NREM sleep. This meant that there had to be active mechanisms, not only for changing from wakefulness to sleep, but also from one type of sleep to another. This implies a balance between arousal and sleep-producing systems, whereby sleep could begin when the overall level of arousal activity falls below that of the sleep-inducing activity. Much remains to be discovered about the centres which induce sleep, but it has been suggested that they are located, like the RAS, in the brain stem below the cerebral cortex. Possibly some of the more selective hypnotic drugs act here, rather than by depressing the RAS.

What regulates these sleep centres remains far from clear, but the processes involved are obviously complex, especially in humans. They must be diffusely linked with many feedback mechanisms via neurons employing various transmitters in a number of physiological pathways. This is apparent from the fact that sleep can be influenced by, for example, hormones (e.g., thyroid hormone), aging, circadian rhythms, mental disease and drugs. Moreover, sleep mechanisms are reflexly linked with certain physiological processes, e.g., respiration, body temperature, muscle relaxation, eye movements and the intensity of environmental light.

However, one transmitter which has been found to be particularly associated with sleep mechanisms is 5-hydroxytryptamine (serotonin; 5-HT). REM sleep has been experimentally induced in humans by administering the amino acid precursor 5-hydroxytryptophan (5-HTP). This crosses the blood-brain barrier and is converted to 5-HT. A drug, parachlorophenylalanine (PCPA), which decreases the body synthesis of 5-HT, reduces the amount of REM sleep with little change in NREM sleep. When PCPA is stopped, REM sleep gradually returns to normal with no rebound increase. Unfortunately, animal studies are more difficult to interpret and suggest that 5-HT influences both NREM and REM sleep.

The precursor of 5-HTP in the body is the essential amino acid L-tryptophan itself, and supplements of this natural substance became popular some years ago as an OTC preparation for a wide range of conditions such as insomnia, mild depression and premenstrual syndrome. It was also administered by responsible psychiatrists for the treatment of depression resistant to the conventional drugs. The relief of insomnia, if genuine, was assumed to be due to the conversion of L-tryptophan to 5-HT in the brain. However, 5-HT can be further metabolized to the pineal hormone melatonin.[4] Brain melatonin synthesis is controlled by external factors, including external light. It has mild hypnotic actions and is known to play a role in the establishment of sleep patterns. OTC preparations containing melatonin have become popular for the treatment of jet lag and other sleep disturbances. It is possible, therefore, that L-tryptophan may act via melatonin rather than via 5-HT itself, though both substances may be involved. OTC melatonin preparations are usually synthetic rather than extracted from animal pineal glands, owing to the dangers of viral contamination and transmission. Their clinical usefulness has still not been adequately verified. Fortunately, they appear to produce few serious side effects.

No problems with L-tryptophan were observed or reported until 1989 when several cases of a bizarre syndrome known as eosinophilia-myalgic syndrome (EMS)[5] occurred in New Mexico, USA. The syndrome led to arthritis, swelling of the feet and hands, rashes, fever, cough and an increase in the eosinophil cells of the blood. On 11 November 1989, the FDA advised against the use of OTC preparations containing L-tryptophan, and by mid-February 1990, after the number of cases of EMS in the USA had risen to 1,269 (including 13 deaths), their sale was banned. In fact, it turned out that the effect was caused by a contaminant in the L-tryptophan, particularly in the preparations put out by a Japanese pharmaceutical firm. In early 1989, this firm began to use a new strain of micro-organism in their fermentation process for L-tryptophan production. Since their L-tryptophan was 99.6% pure, the contaminant, whose chemical structure has now been fairly confidently determined, must be a very potent toxin indeed.

5-HT and melatonin are by no means the only transmitters or hormones thought to be involved in sleep regulation. REM sleep, in particular, would seem to be influenced also by adrenergic mechanisms (noradrenaline and dopamine) and by pathways involving acetylcholine. The cholinergic theory, for example, is consistent with a finding that REM sleep in cats is diminished by atropine and enhanced by physostigmine (eserine), and that these drugs have no effect on NREM sleep. Multiple feedback neurons utilizing a variety of neurotransmitters obviously play a diffuse role in sleep regulating mechanisms. For this reason, probably, a wide range of chemical agents that are able to alter the functions of a number of transmitters can act as hypnotic drugs. For example, barbiturates may inhibit the release of acetylcholine, and benzodiazepines may decrease the tissue metabolism of noradrenaline, dopamine and 5-HT. This does not prove, of course, that these actions are the only ones involved in sleep production. We must remember that serotoninergic, adrenergic and cholinergic pathways in the brain comprise less than 1% of all synaptic connections. This makes it likely that other neurotransmitter systems, some no doubt still to be discovered, play additional roles in sleep regulation.

A question arises: Does the brain itself manufacture an endogenous sleep-inducing substance in the way that it synthesizes its own analgesics? (See Chap. 13, p. 89, on the enkephalins). A recent discovery suggests that this may be so. A group of neuronal membrane proteins has been isolated to which benzodiazepines bind with high affinity, or, in other words, there seem to be brain receptors for benzodiazepines. Just as the detection of morphine-binding receptors in the brain did not imply that morphine itself was the endogenous analgesic, so the findings of benzodiazepine binding sites does not necessarily mean that we synthesize our own natural benzodiazepines. What we do manufacture, if anything, still remains a mystery.

Whatever the neurotransmitter mechanisms involved in sleep, and whether or not we produce our own endogenous hypnotics, we still have much to learn about the biological functions of sleep itself. There is no doubt that REM sleep is important in some way since attempts to suppress it by drugs or other means invariably cause a subsequent compensatory rebound. Claims were made some years ago by an investigator rather appropriately named Dement that depriving subjects of REM sleep, by waking them up every time they showed eye movements, produced temporary psychosis. However, although severe sleep deprivation can certainly cause hallucinations, mental confusion and a progressive deterioration in performance due to lapses in attention, Dement's belief that we need REM sleep to maintain our sanity has not been generally accepted or confirmed. All the same, it is a curious and suggestive fact that acute schizophrenic patients are said not to show a rebound of REM activity after sleep deprivation.

A more recent view, greatly simplified here, is that REM sleep, with its partial arousal and excitation of sensory and motor activity, is responsible for controlling the laying down of long-term memories in the brain, probably as protein molecules. One can imagine the experiences of the day being analyzed and evaluated, and the final conclusions being stored for future reference, a process that one would not be surprised to find associated with dreams. NREM sleep, on the other hand, fits more closely the layman's concept of sleep as a time for the restoration of bodily tissues after a hard day's work. During stages 3 and 4 there is known to be an increase in the release of the growth hormone (somatotrophin) from the pituitary gland, but not during REM sleep. This hormone is important in promoting protein synthesis and raising blood sugar levels, and is necessary for tissue growth and repair.

Ideally, a hypnotic drug should induce normal sleep and not alter the relative proportions of REM and NREM sleep. In the next chapter, we shall discuss how well our existing agents perform this therapeutic task.

27

All the Drowsy Syrups

Macbeth: ... Sleep that knits up the ravell'd sleave of care,
The death of each day's life, sore labour's bath,
Balm of hurt minds, great nature's second course,
Chief nourisher in life's feast ...

W. Shakespeare, *Macbeth*, Act II, Scene 2

The desire to escape the miseries of insomnia by pharmacological means no doubt goes back to prehistoric times, but until the second half of the nineteenth century the only preparations available were herbal in origin. Iago, in Shakespeare's *Othello* (Act III, Scene 3), says:

" ... Not poppy, nor mandragora,
Nor all the drowsy syrups of the world,
Shall ever medicine thee to that sweet sleep
Which thou owedst yesterday."

This suggests that opium and extracts of the root of the mandrake (*Mandragora officinarum*), a solanaceous plant containing alkaloids such as hyoscine, were popular remedies for insomnia at that time. Extracts of *Rauwolfia serpentina* seem to have been used traditionally in India as a hypnotic and it is said that Mahatma Gandhi drank rauwolfia tea as a night-cap. This would, of course, contain the potent alkaloid reserpine. All these agents, morphine, hyoscine and reserpine, are certainly powerful depressants of the central nervous system, but in the pure state would be most unsuitable as hypnotics or sedatives owing to their marked side effects. Alcoholic drinks have been known for a long time, also, and in moderate dosage can be useful mild sedatives and hypnotics, even today, especially for elderly people.

The first laboratory chemical with sleep-inducing properties was chloral hydrate, a chlorine-containing substance related to ethyl alcohol. Synthesized originally in 1832, it came into medical use only in 1869. (Bromides became popular after 1857, but as sedatives rather than hypnotics.) An aqueous solution of chloral hydrate can be taken by mouth, but has a disagreeable taste and may irritate the stomach. This drug is still available today, though little used; and, surprisingly, it is said to cause less suppression of REM sleep and less REM rebound on stopping dosage than later synthetic drugs. However, some tolerance and physical dependence may develop.

More sophisticated synthetic compounds for the treatment of insomnia (and anxiety) had to wait for the twentieth century. The first barbiturate was introduced into medicine in 1903 under the trade name of Veronal. The second, phenobarbitone or Luminal, was developed in 1912 and is still used in the treatment of epilepsy. Since then, more than 2,500 derivatives of barbituric acid have been synthesized, and about 50 have been marketed for clinical application. The barbiturates had a long run for their money, but the search for safer and better hypnotics continued during their reign. The main objections to them were their dangerous side effects, a tendency to produce serious tolerance and dependence and a low therapeutic index. Death may occur from about ten therapeutic doses, so lethal overdosage is only too easy to achieve, either purposely or accidentally. By 1985, only about 9% of hypnotic prescriptions were for barbiturates, and the most commonly selected were the ones with a short to intermediate duration of action ($t_{1/2}$ 14 to 48 hours), e.g., secobarbitone, amobarbitone and pentobarbitone.

The mid-twentieth century search for alternatives to the barbiturates was inclined to be disappointing or even catastrophic. Thalidomide comes to mind as the most disastrous of these, its side effects on the foetus causing an agonizing reappraisal during the 1960s of the control and testing of synthetic drugs (see Chap. 4, p. 38). Meprobamate and glutethimide were more successful, but showed few advantages over the barbiturates. A breakthrough came in 1970 when the drug firm Roche marketed a benzodiazepine derivative flurazepam. Two earlier benzodiazepines, chlordiazepoxide and diazepam (Valium), were already in clinical use as anxiolytics.

So far, the benzodiazepines are probably the nearest approach to the ideal hypnotic (and anxiolytic), but perfection still remains to be achieved. The ideal hypnotic should induce normal sleep and leave the subject refreshed and alert the following morning. In particular, it should not appreciably affect the relative proportions of NREM and REM sleep, though perhaps this is not as serious as was once thought, as Dement's views on the importance of REM sleep are less widely accepted now (see the previous chapter). Excessive dosage should not be toxic or lethal, nor should the drug's toxicity be enhanced by other CNS depressants, e.g., ethyl alcohol. It should not cause tolerance, nor should it lead to any form of dependence or addiction.

At this point, it becomes necessary to explain and define more precisely the terms tolerance, dependence and addiction.[1]

Tolerance implies that repetition of the same dose of a drug gives a reduced pharmacological or therapeutic response, or (to put it another way) a larger dose is required to keep up the same response. There are at least two possible mechanisms for this phenomenon. The enzymes in the liver, or elsewhere, which metabolize the drug, are stimulated to greater activity by the drug itself (*enzyme induction*), and so a higher proportion of the administered drug is destroyed and less remains to act on the brain. This is known as metabolic or pharmacokinetic tolerance. The other mechanism is that the actual cells in the brain become in some way resistant to the drug, and so higher concentrations are needed to produce the equivalent pharmacological activity. This is known as cellular or pharmacodynamic tolerance, and may be caused by reduced efficacy of the receptors.

Dependence on, or habituation to, a drug also takes two forms which must be distinguished: the psychological and the physical. Both forms of dependence are often referred to loosely as *addiction*, and the dependent individual is described as a *drug addict*, but these terms are not officially approved because of their pejorative flavour. In psychological dependence the drug taker becomes enslaved by the pleasant experiences induced by the drug, and comes to regard it as necessary for maintaining an optimal state of mental well-being and satisfaction, and for avoiding feelings of anxiety, tension and unhappiness. Psychological dependence can vary from a mild desire to repeat the dose to severe craving and compulsion, but inability to obtain the drug will not cause actual physical symptoms.

In physical dependence, repeated administration of the drug has led to an alteration in the physiological and biochemical functioning of the cells of the brain, so that, when the drug is stopped, a definite and often intensely unpleasant set of physical symptoms, called the withdrawal or abstinence syndrome, is produced. The subject resorts once again to the drug in order to avoid these agonizing symptoms, since they are *cured* by further dosage.

Physical dependence (the term *neuroadaptation* is sometimes preferred) is a remarkable kind of vicious circle. The neurons react to the biochemical actions of the drug in a homeostatic attempt to restore the *status quo ante*. If we suppose that the action of the drug is to suppress the formation of important neurotransmitters, then the cells would learn to synthesize more of them in order to counteract the effect. If the drug is now withdrawn, the cells are left making abnormally large quantities of transmitters, and this could well have adverse effects on the brain, or on the organism as a whole via the autonomic and endocrine systems. Another possible adaptation could be the synthesis of more transmitter receptor sites on the neurons rather than increased transmitter production itself, but the overall effect would be similar. After a time, however, the altered cells revert to their normal level of function, and the withdrawal symptoms disappear. If tolerance accompanies a liability to physical dependence, then the situation is even more catastrophic. The subject needs to take more and more of the drug in order to maintain a reasonable functional normality of the relevant neurons.

The barbiturates are examples of drugs which produce both types of dependence and both types of tolerance, and this is one of the main reasons for their abandonment by the medical profession (except for inducing anaesthesia and in the treatment of epilepsy). Another reason is their capacity to produce severe depression of respiration and cardiovascular collapse if taken in overdose. This made them popular candidates for suicide attempts.

The benzodiazepines, on the contrary, are less liable to produce fatal respiratory depression, and therefore suicide is said to be virtually impossible with these drugs. However, as with the barbiturates, there is a tendency for ethyl alcohol to potentiate the CNS depressant actions of the benzodiazepines, and the two types of drug should not be combined. Abuse of benzodiazepines seems to be not too serious a problem, though patients on prolonged medication with them do develop psychological dependence. An awareness of their abuse potential has led to some decrease in their popularity since 1973. Nevertheless, benzodiazepines are generally regarded as relatively benign even in acute overdosage, as compared with all other classes of hypnotics. One possible reason for this may be related to a unique feature of their mode of action. It is now thought that benzodiazepines are able to potentiate the actions of a neuro-inhibitory transmitter known as gamma-aminobutyric acid (GABA), and that most, if not all, of their hypnotic activity is based on this. Such a mechanism would place a limit on the CNS depressant properties of the benzodiazepines, since they would depend on the release of an endogenous inhibitory neurotransmitter (GABA).

The use of benzodiazepines, however, is not free of some of the other disadvantages of hypnotic therapy. One of these is the so-called *hangover effect*. A drug taken at bedtime in sufficient dosage to induce a good night's sleep will not, for obvious pharmacokinetic reasons, cease to act as soon as the subject gets up in the morning. A certain proportion of the original dose is bound to remain in the body and carry over into the afternoon. This will cause some residual drowsiness and possible impairment of mental and motor skills. The situation can be improved by choosing the smallest dose necessary to ensure adequate rest, and by selecting a drug with a short half-life $(t_{1/2})$. However, the half-life of a drug may be prolonged in older patients.

It will be remembered that the half-life (see Chap. 12, p. 87) is the time required to remove, either by metabolism or excretion or both, half the administered dose of the drug from the body. The benzodiazepines triazolam (Halcion) and temazepam (Restoril), for example, have $t_{1/2}$s of 1.5–5 hours and 9 hours respectively and are most suitable as hypnotics. For the treatment of anxiety states, on the other hand, the longer acting benzodiazepines are preferable, e.g., diazepam (Valium, $t_{1/2}$ 24–48 hours), flurazepam (Dalmane, $t_{1/2}$ 47–100 hours) and lorazepam (Ativan, $t_{1/2}$ 10–20 hours). The three most prescribed benzodiazepines in 1985 were flurazepam, triazolam and temazepam.

Even the shorter-acting benzodiazepines, however, do not obviate the possibility of a hangover effect the following day, since small amounts of the drug will continue to circulate in the blood stream. Of course, one could hope that, after an improved night's sleep, the subject's alertness and mental functioning might be better than it would have been after a night tortured by insomnia, even if some drug does remain in the body. Unfortunately, there is little evidence that relieving insomnia by administering these drugs necessarily improves alertness; it may, in fact, impair it. A 1983 study of general practice patients in Britain found that when taking benzodiazepines they had more car accidents than when drug-free, and other investigations have confirmed this effect on driving skills and on cognitive performance in general. And, to make matters more confusing, it appears that good sleepers and hypnotic-free insomniacs show no significant difference in performance when given tests of cognitive function!

There has also been a growing concern in recent years that even the benzodiazepines can produce withdrawal disturbances, implying some degree of physical dependence.[2] This seems to be more noticeable with the newer, short-acting agents. Another recent, and more serious, scare has been associated specifically with the popular drug triazolam (Halcion), which has been shown to cause depression, bizarre behaviour, paranoia, hallucinations and short-term memory loss. The banning of this drug in Britain is referred to in Chap. 6, p. 49. In that country, the *British Medical Journal* reported in 1992[3] that a convict who stabbed a fellow prison inmate 17 times after drinking tea containing triazolam was acquitted of attempted murder. This was the first British case to cite the mental side effects of this drug in a legal defence. Perhaps as a result, the pharmaceutical firm Upjohn has offerred in the USA to defend and indemnify those doctors who prescribe Halcion and are subsequently sued by patients claiming personal injury from the hypnotic.

The truth is that, until we know more about the basic neurochemistry of sleep and sedation, our search for the safe hypnotic and anxiolytic with selective activities is but a fumbling in the dark. Perhaps the ultimate breakthrough will come with the identification in the brain of the naturally occurring sleep-inducing substances (if they exist), along the lines of the naturally analgesic enkephalins. In the meantime, the more we can dispense with the use of synthetic hypnotic drugs the better, especially for those over 60.

28

The Conquest of Pain?

> But pain is perfect miserie, the worst
> Of evils, and, excessive, overturnes
> All patience ...
>
> John Milton (1608–1674), *Paradise Lost*, Book 6

Greater than the human desire to relieve insomnia is the desire to avoid pain and suffering, and the fear of pain and suffering. Yet, like sleep, pain has necessary biological functions. It is the way our bodies inform us that something is wrong. It warns us of the dangers of fire, sharp objects, poisons and caustic irritants, and encourages us to rest when we are sick or injured. Unfortunately, for a variety of reasons, pain may become chronic and persist beyond its immediate function as a warning signal. Chronic pain can play havoc with the sufferer's way of life, his relationships with others, and his work. His personality may be seriously affected, leading to depression, withdrawal and ultimate despair. Continuous or recurrent pain is estimated to affect almost 19% of the population of the USA, or more than 50 million people.[1]

Pain sensation is conveyed to the brain via neurons that begin as free nerve endings in the skin and other bodily tissues and organs. These nerve endings respond to harmful stimuli, e.g., extreme heat or cold, pressure and mechanical injury. They also respond to certain chemical substances such as histamine or bradykinin, which are released from inflamed or injured tissues. The nerve impulses so produced travel to the spinal cord where they form synapses with ascending nerve tracts there. These tracts lead to the brain and terminate at a structure known as the thalamus, where the pain sensations are processed by being passed on to other structures. These evaluate what sort of pain it is, how intense, where it is located and what to do about it.

Pain impulses from the periphery are transmitted by two systems involving fibres of different sizes, smaller ones called A-Delta which conduct rapidly, and larger C-fibres which conduct more slowly. The immediate sharp pain following an injury travels along the A-delta fibres, and draws attention to the causative agent so that measures to avoid it can be taken. The delayed pain mediated by the C-fibres, typically a dull ache, maintains attention and so encourages one to look after the injured part and prevent or minimize permanent damage.

In order to reduce or prevent painful sensation, it is necessary to block its origin and transmission at the various sites outlined above. These are: (1) at the peripheral nerve endings, either directly or by an inhibitory action on the release of pain-producing substances from the surrounding tissues; (2) along the pain fibres travelling to the spinal cord; and (3) in the central nervous system itself. In recent years it has been suggested that there is a fourth site in the spinal cord, and perhaps in the brain too, where other forms of sensory stimuli can compete with, and thereby help suppress, pain transmission. Such stimuli, e.g., heat, cold, massage, have formed the basis of the physical treatment of pain from time immemorial. They work by a process of *counterirritation*, and are thought to close *gates* in the spinal cord and brain, preventing onward transmission of pain. This mechanism may involve certain neurotransmitters including the enkephalins (see Chap. 13, p. 93 and later).

This *Gate Theory* has also been invoked to explain the apparent efficacy of acupuncture in relieving certain types of pain. The Chinese, who have for centuries utilized this technique of inserting fine needles into precisely defined sites in the skin and underlying tissues known as *acupuncture points*, explained their successes in terms of promoting the flow of a *vital force* (*ch'i*) through a postulated system of ducts or channels (*meridians*). These meridians were supposed to link up with the various organs of the body, but modern anatomists have not been able to detect their presence with any certainty. This is perhaps a further example of how a treatment found to be effective in traditional medicine came to be explained by fanciful, armchair theories. After all, the systematic experimental study of human anatomy only began with Vesalius in the sixteenth century. Acupuncturists claim not only to relieve pain, but also to cure or alleviate many diseases. It is usual nowadays to improve the therapy by twirling the needles gently or by passing electrical impulses through them.

Acupuncture has been known to, and even practiced by, some Western physicians since about the eighteenth century, but it became something of a cult in the 1970s when the Mao Zedong régime in China publicized it as a method of anaesthesia during certain surgical operations. Visiting Western surgeons were shown various procedures, e.g., thyroid removal, performed allegedly without the use of analgesics or anaesthetics. When it was revealed some years later that many of these demonstrations were fraudulent, and that drugs *were* used, the enthusiasm of Western doctors for acupuncture cooled considerably. Much research has been carried out by neurophysiologists and neuroanatomists, and it soon became clear that, although acupuncture may indeed reduce pain, this relief can still be obtained even if the needles are inserted at randomly chosen sites, rather than at the traditional points. The present view is that much still remains to be understood about why acupuncture works in some patients (though not all), but some physiologists believe that the procedure acts through the release of enkephalins. Critics of this view regard the underlying mechanism as more likely to be based on the phenomenon of counterirritation. The well-known efficacy of percutaneous electrical stimulation in helping to relieve temporarily deep (visceral) pain is also thought to be due to counterirritation. Another technique known as moxibustion, in which the dried leaves of certain plants are burned on the skin, was also popular in traditional Chinese medicine. Since this causes scarification and pain, the role of counterirritation in this procedure is easy to accept!

Physical therapies, including acupuncture, provide relatively ineffective relief of pain, and most of us prefer to take advantage of the various types of analgesic drugs, in spite of their inevitable toxicity. The two most important and widely used categories of analgesics are the non-narcotics for mild to moderate pain, and the narcotics or opioids for more serious pain, especially that arising from disease or injury in the visceral organs. In addition, there are the local and general anaesthetics which can temporarily eliminate pain during surgical procedures and in dentistry.

Most of the non-narcotic analgesics possess a variable capacity to suppress tissue inflammation, and so these agents are often known as non-steroidal anti-inflammatory drugs, or NSAIDs for short. Non-steroidal refers to the fact that they are not chemically related to steroids, some of which, e.g., cortisone or hydrocortisone, also have anti-inflammatory properties. They may also show antipyretic activity, i.e., they lower a raised body temperature and so relieve a fever. This is a central nervous system action on the body's thermostat in the hypothalamus. Their analgesic effects, however, occur mainly at the peripheral sites of origin of the pain in the tissues. It is possible that some of these drugs, especially acetaminophen (Tylenol), can also moderate pain perception in the CNS itself.

Among the NSAIDs, the salicylates have been known and utilized for centuries in various cultures since they occur in a number of plants, e.g., the bark of the willow tree (*Salix alba*). However, the active principle, salicin, was not isolated until 1829 when it was shown to be salicylic alcohol combined with glucose. Salicylic alcohol can be easily converted to sodium salicylate and, in 1875, this was employed for the treatment of rheumatic fever and as an antipyretic. It also turned out later to be valuable in the treatment of gout by promoting the removal of uric acid which accumulates in gouty joints. The acetyl derivative of salicylic acid was first synthesized in 1853, but it remained on the laboratory shelf until 1899 when it was introduced into medicine by the drug firm Bayer under the trade name of Aspirin. This has become probably the most widely used drug of all times and its name is no longer the property of Bayer but has found its way into the dictionaries of many languages. D.R. Laurence reported in his 1980 edition of *Clinical Pharmacology*[2] that the British eat about 2,000 tons of aspirin yearly, or two tablets every week for the total population of the country. By 1990, the USA was said to be consuming 10, 000–20,000 tons annually. The recent recommendation that we exploit the anticoagulant action of the drug by ingesting regular small (85mg) doses (baby aspirins) as a prophylaxis against the threat of heart attacks and strokes, and possibly other conditions, is likely to increase its popularity.

It is strange that the mechanism of the analgesic action of a drug used so widely and for so long remained a mystery until as recently as 1971. In that year, John Vane, working at the Wellcome Laboratories in London, showed that aspirin and a closely related NSAID indomethacin influenced the formation and actions in tissues of substances known as autacoids. Autocoids are chemicals normally present or readily formed in tissue cells which can produce a wide range of pharmacological actions when released locally, e.g., in response to injury. They probably play an important physiological role in tissue healing and repair. Histamine and bradykinin are typical autacoids (see p. 193) that can stimulate pain by a direct effect on the nerve endings. Others, known as prostaglandins, are released from inflamed tissues and also have some degree of pain-producing activity. More importantly, in this connection, they can also sensitize the nerve endings to the actions of the other pain-producing autacoids. In effect, the prostaglandins are acting as an amplification system for the pain mechanism. Vane and his coworkers found that aspirin and indomethacin could inhibit an enzyme responsible for the biosynthesis of prostaglandins, and so reduce their levels in the tissues. This removes one contributory factor to the pain mechanism, and may also eliminate part of the inflammatory process. For this discovery, John Vane received the Nobel Prize for Medicine and Physiology in 1982.[3]

Local anaesthetics, such as procaine (Novocain) or lignocaine (Xylocaine), act directly on the pain fibres (site 2 above) by altering their permeability to certain ions, e.g., sodium. This prevents further transmission of the nerve impulses along the fibre. Many of the local anaesthetics in use today are based structurally on the alkaloid cocaine, which occurs in the South American plant *Erythroxylon coca*, chewed by Bolivian and Peruvian Indians to stave off tiredness in the high Andes. The plant was brought to Europe in the nineteenth century, and in 1858 the alkaloid was isolated and purified in the laboratory of the German chemist Friedrich Wöhler.[4] Wöhler noted that the substance applied to the tongue caused a temporary numbness. This led in time to the use of cocaine as a local anaesthetic by injection, but it was soon realized that this agent had marked side effects and a capacity to induce serious addiction (see p. 139 for Freud's experiments with cocaine).

The use of general anaesthetic agents to eliminate the pain, and also the awareness, of traumatic surgical operations was developed in the USA and the UK during the 1840s, against much opposition from religious groups.[5] These agents are mostly volatile substances such as nitrous oxide, diethyl ether, halothane and ketamine. They are breathed in by the subject and absorbed through the lungs into the blood stream. From the blood they reach the brain where they exert their actions. General anaesthesia may also be produced by the injection of certain non-volatile lipid-soluble substances, e.g., barbiturates such as thiopentone, and the recently developed phenol derivative propofol.

But one of the most powerful of analgesic agents, opium from the poppy plant *Papaver somniferum*, has been known to mankind since prehistoric times. The ancient Sumerians (4,000 B.C.) had an ideograph for the poppy, meaning joy plant. Sites of the Stone Age lake dwellers in Switzerland, who lived about 4,000 years ago, have revealed seeds and the large seed heads of the cultivated poppy. Egypt may have been the first civilization to use the opium poppy for medical purposes, and from there it spread to Asia Minor and further afield. A reference to poppy juice is found in the writings of the Greek philosopher Theophrastus (370–287 B.C); opium is derived from the Greek word for juice. Later, Arabian physicians became experienced in the medical applications of opium, and found it particularly efficacious for the treatment of dysentery. In Europe, Paracelsus is said to have introduced an alcoholic extract, or tincture, of opium known as laudanum, and this preparation came to be widely used by the sixteenth century. The identification and purification of the main active principle in opium, morphine, and the determination of its complete chemical structure, have been described in Chap. 2 (p. 20 et seq.).

The analgesic activity of morphine is on the central nervous system and, as explained in Chap. 13 (p. 93), it acts by imitating the naturally occurring brain enkephalins. It also has many other actions and affects many systems in the body, e.g., it depresses respiration and the cough reflex, constricts the pupil of the eye and causes severe constipation. Some of these actions may on occasion be useful medicinally, but when morphine is given for pain relief they become unwanted side effects. The most undesirable feature of morphine's pharmacology, of course, is its capacity to induce tolerance, addiction and a withdrawal syndrome.

The first attempt to convert morphine to a substance devoid of unwanted actions was made in 1874 at St. Mary's Hospital in London. This was heroin, the acetylated derivative, and in 1898 it was introduced as a remedy for cough and to cure morphine addiction. Heroin appeared to be most efficacious for both these conditions, but several years passed before it was realized that the *cured* addicts were only substituting one drug of abuse for another. In fact, heroin is even more disastrously addictive than morphine, probably because it crosses to the brain across the blood-brain barrier better than morphine. It has no place in modern medical practice, except perhaps for terminal cancer patients, but it is one of the most destructive and dangerous of the illegal drugs of abuse in the world today.

Since the 1930s, a large number of semi-synthetic agents with morphine-like activity have been developed. The earliest of these were pethidine (UK) or meperidine (USA) (Demerol, 1939) and methadone (Dolophine, 1945); other, more recent, ones are oxymorphone (Numorphan), levorphanol (Levo-Dromoran) and the relatively mild propoxyphene (Darvon). These may have some advantages over morphine, but they still cause marked tolerance and physical dependence, and so are undesirable for general use as analgesics. It seemed impossible to dissociate the two actions, the analgesic and the addictive, until, in the

1950s, hopes were raised when it was discovered that certain semi-synthetic derivatives of the opium alkaloids possessed a surprising pharmacological property.

The first important member of this group of drugs was nalorphine, and it was found to reverse the actions of the opiates and opioids. A patient in a coma and with severely depressed breathing, due to morphine overdose, recovered consciousness and showed improved respiration following an injection of the drug. Chemically, nalorphine is N-allylnormorphine, the full name indicating that a methyl group (CH_3) on a nitrogen atom in the morphine molecule has been replaced by another group known as the allyl radical (C_3H_5). Nalorphine not only reverses the actions of morphine, but can also precipitate the typical withdrawal symptoms in a narcotic addict. The main application of the latter property is not for the detection of addicts (though this has been unkindly done in the past), but in animal tests. New narcotic analgesics can be checked quickly for *abuse potential* (i.e., a liability to cause physical dependence) by administering nalorphine after a few doses of the new agent.

Later, some curious facts about the actions of nalorphine came to light.[6] It is quite a powerful analgesic when given on its own, but its capacity to diminish the depth and rate of breathing is much less than that of morphine. It acts as an antagonist to morphine because it has a stronger affinity for the morphine receptors, but a weaker activity on the centres controlling respiration in the brain stem. Nalorphine, therefore, displaces a previously administered dose of morphine from its receptors, and substitutes its own weaker activity on the respiratory centres. The subject recovers, at least until the nalorphine effect wears off, because of the marked improvement in his respiration. As explained in Chap. 13 (p. 93), such a drug is known as a partial agonist. Complete antagonists to opioids have also been developed, namely naloxone (Narcan) and naltrexone (Trexan), which strongly displace morphine, heroin, etc. from the receptors, but then exert no action of their own at all. These drugs are clearly safer and more effective antidotes for opioid overdosage, and nowadays have replaced nalorphine for that purpose.

However, nalorphine has continued to arouse interest among pharmacologists because it produces a number of unexpected effects not shared by morphine or heroin. These are unpleasant feelings of malaise, anxiety and mental disturbance, i.e., a dysphoria quite the opposite to the marked euphoria or happiness induced by the addictive opioids. This suggests, and recent research has confirmed it, that there are several types of narcotic receptors in the central nervous system, possibly at least three known as mu, kappa and delta (see p. 94). Presumably nalorphine exerts its dysphoric actions on those receptors which are little affected by morphine.

Since nalorphine possesses reasonably good pain-killing properties, and the dysphoria it induces might be expected to diminish its attractiveness as a drug of abuse, the exciting idea arose that it could be the long-sought-after non-addictive opiate. Unfortunately, the dysphoria is so disagreeable that many patients are reluctant to take the drug and seem to prefer the untreated pain. Moreover, nalorphine *can* actually cause tolerance, physical dependence and a withdrawal syndrome, showing that addiction does not necessarily require the prior existence of euphoria. But the hunt was on, and in recent years a wide range of partial agonists and mixed agonist-antagonists has been introduced. The aim, of course, is to find one that is a potent analgesic, yet causes some dysphoria but not too much.

Two drugs which once seemed promising as substitutes for morphine are pentazocin (Talwin) and buprenorphine (Buprenex), but these are far from perfect. Buprenorphine is a semisynthetic opioid derived from thebaine (another poppy alkaloid with negligible analgesic activity), but it also causes dysphoric symptoms such as nausea, dizziness, sweating and headache. Addiction to buprenophine and pentazocine is also seen, though the abuse potential is said to be much reduced. Newer synthetic drugs are fentanyl and alfentanil. Fentanyl, a μ-agonist, is 80 times more potent than morphine, but has a shorter duration of action (one to two hours). Alfentanil is related chemically to fentanyl, but has only one-third the potency and is even shorter acting; it has been approved for use in general anaesthesia (GA).

Other drugs useful in GA are α_2-blockers such as clonidine and its relative dexmedetomidine. Clonidine and its congeners were originally developed to treat high blood pressure, but it was found that when administered together with certain GAs it became possible to reduce GA dosage and still produce adequate anaesthesia. The α_2-blockers can also induce anaesthesia by themselves.[7]

The mid-1970s saw a completely different, and seemingly more promising, approach to the problem of finding a truly non-addictive narcotic analgesic. It was then that Kosterlitz and Hughes in Aberdeen, Scotland, isolated the natural analgesics of the brain, the enkephalins (see Chap. 13, p. 93). These endogenous substances, as we mentioned, show little obvious chemical resemblance to morphine itself. They are pentapeptides, consisting of a chain of five amino acids, and the first two recognized were methionine-enkephalin and leucine-enkephalin, differing only in one amino acid. Since they occur naturally in the brain and act presumably as neurotransmitters at opiate receptors, addiction was not expected to be one of their side effects following clinical use.

Unfortunately, these agents were immediately found to be quire unsuitable for clinical application. On administration, they did not remain in the circulation long enough to cross the blood-brain barrier and enter the central nervous system. Polypeptides like the enkephalins are extremely rapidly broken down in the body by enzymes called peptidases, and it was soon discovered that enkephalins injected into animals disappeared from the circulation within a minute. The drug companies, who were naturally very excited at the prospect of reaping a bonanza from these new compounds, worked hard to modify their chemical structures so that they were not attacked by the tissue peptidases; and also to produce more lipid-soluble analogues that would better penetrate the brain. Perhaps the closest approach to success was achieved by Sandoz, who designed an enkephalin analogue FK-33824[8] which acted powerfully on opiate receptors and was extremely resistant to enzyme destruction. This compound produced analgesia when injected directly into the brains of mice, and was 30,000 times more potent than enkephalin itself.

When FK-33824 was tested clinically in human volunteers, a number of disconcerting effects were observed. Very small doses caused a sense of heaviness in the limbs and chest — *but* no analgesia. Higher doses were tried, but the peripheral effects became so disagreeable that the clinical trials had to be stopped. Even more discouraging was the finding that these synthetic enkephalins did, after all, lead to tolerance, addiction and withdrawal symptoms.

The drug firms abandoned their attempts to make (and patent) the ideal non-addictive analgesic; and one can even feel a little sorry for them as they must have put a lot of capital into these efforts without gaining any profit whatsoever. (Of course, they can cover their losses in such ventures by increasing the price of their successful new drugs.)

It was then realized that the reason why the brain does not develop tolerance and addiction to its own natural enkephalins is that these agents, like most neurotransmitters, are rapidly broken down by special enzymes close to the receptors. Tolerance and addiction only develop if the substance (e.g., morphine) is in contact with its receptors for a prolonged period of time; and this is what happens with a stable analogue like FK-33824.

So here we have a classical Catch-22 situation. An unstable drug will not reach the desired site of action, and a stable one is bound to cause addiction. Obviously, the Holy Grail of a perfect non-addictive narcotic analgesic with no unpleasant peripheral or central side effects still eludes us.

29

Addiction: The Ecstasy and the Agony

> I took it [tincture of opium] and in an hour, O heavens!
> What a revulsion! What a resurrection, from its lower
> depths, of the inner spirit! That my pain had vanished
> was now a trifle in my eyes; this negative effect was
> swallowed up in the immensity of those positive effects
> which had opened before me, in the abyss of divine
> enjoyment thus suddenly revealed.
>
> Thomas de Quincey, in
> *Confessions of an English Opium Eater* (1821)

A 1981 report from the United Nations Narcotics Control Agency claimed that drug abuse was on the rise worldwide, with addicts becoming younger and turning to stronger drugs increasingly easy to obtain. Addiction, they said, was growing for all drugs: opium and heroin, cocaine, cannabis (marijuana), as well as for amphetamines and other synthetic agents.

Is the situation any better today? In the USA, during the Reagan and Bush administrations, a much publicized war on drugs was waged at enormous financial cost, but the results were far from spectacular. By 1989, it seemed that some drugs had become less popular (e.g., the hallucinogens), and others had peaked in street popularity (e.g., phencyclidine (PCP or Angel Dust) and cocaine). The overall use of *recreational* drugs had, in general, levelled off or even decreased slightly, but The National Foundation for Brain Research in Washington D.C. reported in 1992 that alcohol abuse still cost the US $40 billion, and abuse of other drugs $71 billion per year. These enormous sums include the direct cost of medical care as well as indirect costs, such as lost wages and impaired productivity, and represent up to 7.3% of the nation's Gross Domestic Product. Obviously, the problem remains a serious one. But before commenting further on this, we must describe and define in some detail the various ways in which drug abuse and drug addiction can manifest themselves.

It should now be clear to the reader that, although drugs have their necessary uses, they are all too commonly misused, over-used and incompetently used. The blame for this can be laid at various doors, for example, the medical profession itself with its inadequate training in pharmacology, and the pharmaceutical industry with its ruthless commercialism. But in drug *abuse*, it is the consumer himself or herself who creates the problem by his or her own ill-advised self-medication.

Drug abuse has been carefully defined, therefore, as the "self-administration of any drug in a manner which deviates from approved medical or social patterns within a given culture". The reference here to social patterns and the cultural background indicates that this whole problem is not purely a pharmacological one, but must be evaluated in a much wider context. It is this fact, perhaps, which is responsible for the sharp differences of opinion among experts in this field.

Drug abuse is not confined strictly to agents acting on the central nervous system. The person who is so concerned about his colonic performance that he feels the constant need to take medication to ensure *bowel regularity* could be said to abuse laxatives. However, drug abuse usually implies the harmful self-administration of the so-called psychotropic agents, and it is these in particular which can cause the most serious social and personal problems. The important reason for this is that many (but not all) of the drugs acting on the central nervous system can induce biochemical changes in the functioning of the brain cells which lead to pharmacodynamic (cellular) tolerance, and to psychological and physical dependence.

The mechanisms of cellular tolerance to, and physical dependence on, psychotropic drugs are almost certainly related in some way not yet fully understood to neurotransmitter production and balance in the brain. A simple model for these effects was outlined in Chap. 27 (p. 190), in connection with the hypnotic and anxiolytic drugs. The development of a compulsive need for a drug of addiction is, therefore, physiological in origin, implicit in all of us, and is not a result of weak personality or lack of moral fibre. This is confirmed by the fact that other mammals can, under laboratory conditions, become addicted to much the same range of drugs that appeals to *Homo sapiens*. However, in humans social factors obviously play an important role in determining whether a particular individual will risk experimentation with addictive drugs. These factors are: availability, curiosity, influence of peer groups, general social acceptability, attitudes towards authority and, no doubt, many others.

A 1964 WHO Committee on Addiction-Producing Drugs defined drug dependence as "a state arising from repeated administration of a drug on a periodic or continuous basis". Dependence can be classified for convenience according to the types of drug involved. These are: opioids, barbiturates, ethyl alcohol, anaesthetic gases, local anaesthetics, volatile solvents, central stimulants, phencyclidine (PCP), nicotine and caffeine. These different drug groups show varying patterns of tolerance and dependence, and some of the more important ones will now be discussed.

The *opioid-type* of dependence occurs with the analgesic alkaloids of the opium poppy, i.e., morphine and codeine, and with their synthetic and semi-synthetic analogues, e.g., heroin, pethidine, methadone. All these drugs have been so extremely valuable in the relief of severe pain (see Chap. 28, p. 197) that no doctor, as the great physicians of the past used to say, could bear to contemplate the practice of medicine without them. Unfortunately, these drugs are the ones most potent in producing tolerance and physical dependence.

Morphine addicts may need eventually to take 20 to 30 times the normal analgesic dose (10–20 milligrams) in order to experience the usual gratifying response. Authenticated cases of addicts injecting 5 grams daily have been recorded, a dose considerably in excess of the lethal one for a non-addicted (or *naive*) subject.

Physical dependence is also strikingly exemplified by the narcotic analgesics; 80–90% of the subjects who inject themselves with heroin in a non-medical environment will become physically dependent on the drug, and will need repeated *fixes* in order to prevent the development of the extremely disagreeable withdrawal or abstinence symptoms. These withdrawal effects can also be demonstrated in experimental animals such as rats and mice. Since these drugs are the ones that broadly depress the central nervous system, the withdrawal symptoms not surprisingly manifest themselves as a *rebound hyperexcitability* or *hyperstimulation* of the CNS.

The first symptoms of withdrawal are noticed about the time the next dose would have been due, and represents what is called *purposive behaviour*. This is purely psychological, and is an attempt to persuade someone to provide more drug through demands, pleas and complaints of intolerable pain.

True physical or *non-purposive* symptoms, over which the addict has no control, begin about 8–12 hours after the last dose. These are runny eyes and nose (lacrimation and rhinorhoea), yawning and sweating. At 12–14 hours, he may fall into a tossing, restive sleep (the *yen*) for several hours, and then wake in a miserable state with dilated pupils, loss of appetite, gooseflesh and tremors. The peak of the syndrome appears after about 48–72 hours of abstinence, with insomnia, violent yawning, nausea, vomiting and diarrhoea. Hyperactivity of the muscles makes the skin hairs stand on end, and leads to an appearance fancifully compared to that of a plucked turkey. This is the origin of the expression *cold turkey treatment*, used to describe the process of curing an opium addict by abrupt withdrawal of the drug. Severe abdominal cramps and very painful muscle spasms (origin of the phrase *kicking the habit*) complete the dismal picture.

Many of the symptoms of withdrawal are obviously related to overactivity of the sympathetic and parasympathetic divisions of the autonomic nervous system (ANS), and of certain other centres in the brain. This can certainly be attributed, at least in part, to abnormalities in neurotransmitter production by the opioid-conditioned neurons of the CNS, as mentioned above. However, in spite of considerable research, we still do not know what are the actual transmitters or other neurochemicals involved in this rebound hyperexcitability, though noradrenaline, acetylcholine, dopamine, serotonin (5-HT), histamine and others have been suggested for this role. It is not unlikely that several of these play a part in the overall picture. Presumably they are the same transmitters that play a part in the analgesic and other actions of the opioids, and, one may add, in the actions of the enkephalins.

Like morphine, the barbiturates and ethyl alcohol also produce an overall depression of the central nervous system (CNS), and cause tolerance and both psychological and physical dependence. Less is known, however, about the biochemistry of these processes in those two groups, but the withdrawal symptoms show features in common, suggesting certain similarities in the underlying mechanisms. This is further supported by the existence of cross-tolerance, i.e., a subject made tolerant to barbiturates becomes automatically tolerant to alcohol, and vice versa.

Withdrawal symptoms with barbiturates and alcohol can be severe and unpleasant, and are characterized, as expected, by rebound hyper-excitability. The syndrome with alcohol has acquired the special name of *delirium tremens*; the addict shows anxiety, vomiting, tremors, sweating, increase of blood pressure and insomnia. He may become delirious, experiencing hallucinations, and develop epileptic seizures. Barbiturate withdrawal is similar, but the epileptic convulsions tend to be more intense, and may be fatal.

Barbiturates now have little place in modern medical practice, but alcohol, which is, of course, a socially acceptable drug of abuse, is still a major scourge. Alcohol remains the single most important drug of abuse in European, North American and other Western-style communities. Nevertheless, the problem, serious though it is, is less so than it might be, since only about 5–7% of alcohol-takers eventually become addicted, and the condition may take three to ten years to develop. The comparable figures for barbiturates are similar, 5–10%; for morphine and for heroin they are 80–90%.

The two most potent *stimulant* drugs of abuse, amphetamine (and its analogues)[1] and cocaine, present a rather different picture. Tolerance to these drugs tends to be slight, as with amphetamine, or possibly absent, as with cocaine, when taken in moderate dosage. Psychological dependence on amphetamine can be severe, but cocaine is less compulsive to the devotee who claims to be able to "take it or leave it".

The question of physical dependence and withdrawal syndrome with these stimulants has generated much controversy, partly because there is considerable disagreement about the basic facts. Some authorities deny that they produce these effects at all, but perhaps the reason is that, since the drugs are stimulants, withdrawal symptoms would be expected to show a rebound hypoexcitability. Addicts would, therefore, tend to demonstrate apathy, sedation, deep sleep and other manifestations of severe depression of the CNS. This would not cause the subject any marked degree of discomfort; he would merely *sleep it off* until his central neurons recovered normal excitability.

For example, when the chronic amphetamine user stops taking the drug, he experiences fatigue and depression (and this may be to the point of suicide), and after long periods of intoxication he may lapse into coma for a day. Withdrawal from cocaine seems to occur in a series of phases. During the first nine hours to 14 days, the addict experiences intense craving and cocaine-seeking behaviour (*the crash*). Associated with this phase are feelings of intense agitation, depression and decreased appetite, leading to fatigue, insomnia and exhaustion. Finally, the appetite rebounds and there is a need to sleep.

In fact it is the continued long-term dosage with these two stimulants which leads to hyperexcitability and dangerous euphoria, and the development of socially unacceptable behaviour. This is presumably caused by over-stimulation of the sympathetic nervous system. Amphetamine is, of course, a sympathomimetic drug, imitating the actions of adrenaline and noradrenaline; and cocaine acts in a similar way by preventing the re-uptake of catecholamines at the nerve endings (see p. 164 in connection with tricyclic antidepressants). Eventually the chronic addict exhibits symptoms closely resembling those of paranoid schizophrenia, with delusions of being influenced, ideas of reference, and visual and auditory hallucinations. Other psychotic manifestations are stereotyped searching and examining movements. The addict seems to enjoy repetitive dismantling of objects like watches or TV sets; he may start picking at his skin under the impression that minute parasites are hidden there.

In view of the devastating effects of addiction to amphetamine and cocaine, it is reasonable that the recreational use of these drugs is socially condemned and legally outlawed. There are, however, central stimulants of a milder nature, but society tends to be somewhat irrational about their legal status. Drinking caffeine-containing coffee, tea or Coca-Cola, for example, carries no stigma. Tobacco is still legal, but its use meets increasing social disapproval, especially in public places. The smoking of cannabis (marijuana) is arguably less harmful to one's health in the long run than tobacco-smoking, but remains an illegal activity.

Caffeine is a member of a group of substances known as xanthines, three of which occur in popular beverages. Tea contains caffeine and theophylline, cocoa caffeine and theobromine, and coffee provides only caffeine. Caffeine is the most centrally stimulant of the three, and in excess can cause feelings of tension and anxiety, tremors, insomnia and irregularities of the heart beat (extrasystoles). A slight degree of tolerance to its effects may occur, and coffee drinkers who imbibe five or more cups a day, and then stop, may experience some withdrawal symptoms, e.g., headache and irritability. But caffeine is a relatively harmless drug with no conclusive evidence of long-term deleterious effects.

Nicotine addiction is quite a different story. As mentioned in Chap. 18 (p. 128), this substance has widespread pharmacological actions in the body through a stimulant (and later a depressant) effect on all sympathetic and parasympathetic ganglia. It occurs in the tobacco plant *Nicotiana tabacum* which has been smoked, chewed or applied externally as a salve by American Indians for many centuries, and was brought to Europe following the voyages of Christopher Columbus in the 1490s. Nicotine might be considered not too dangerous a drug as it is a less powerful stimulant than amphetamine or cocaine. It is the popular route of administration by inhaling the smoke of the burning tobacco leaf that is the problem. It is estimated that approximately 4,000 different compounds are generated by this process. These are classified into two groups, the gaseous and the particulate. The gaseous phase contains such undesirable and toxic substances as carbon monoxide, nitrogen oxides, ammonia, hydrogen cyanide and many others. The particulate matter, or tar, is known to contain substances that can cause cancerous changes in the body tissues. Since roughly 26% of adult Americans still smoke (mainly cigarettes), it is not surprising that about 350,000 smokers die every year from the toxic effects of tobacco. The total cost of smoking-related health care and lost productivity is approximately $65 billion per year. Some of the major health risks of chronic smoking are: cancer, especially of the lung; an increased tendency to suffer strokes and heart attacks; and respiratory problems such as bronchitis and emphysema. Since smoking is a social activity and the burning tip of the cigarette releases a similar range of toxic compounds into the surrounding atmosphere, those who do not smoke are also at risk (so-called *passive smoking* which, according to a former US Surgeon General, kills more than 50,000 American non-smokers a year).

In this chapter, however, we are concerned primarily with the role of nicotine as a drug of addiction. The average cigarette contains about 10mg of nicotine, and about 1–2 mg of this reaches the lungs during smoking and is readily absorbed. The drug crosses the blood-brain barrier and acts on central cholinergic receptors. The *naive* smoker tends to suffer nausea, vomiting and dizziness, but tolerance soon develops to these actions. On the cardiovascular system, nicotine increases the blood pressure and the strength of the heart contractions. Adrenaline and noradrenaline are released from the adrenal glands, and there is a decrease in muscle tone leading to a feeling of relaxation and tranquillity. The brain is directly stimulated, causing changes in the electroencephalogram (EEG) and a sense of euphoria. Smokers have been shown to perform better on some cognitive tasks than when deprived of cigarettes.

The physical dependence on nicotine is much more intense than used to be thought. When the pure drug is given intravenously to volunteers, it is found to be more addicting than cocaine, and is responsible for a marked abstinence or withdrawal syndrome somewhat similar to that produced by cocaine and amphetamines. The syndrome in smokers occurs within hours of stopping smoking, and manifests itself as decreased heart rate, restlessness, drowsiness, inability to concentrate, irritability and feelings of hostility. There may be problems of sleeping, with alterations in the patterns of REM sleep. Symptoms are worst during the first week of abstinence and decrease over a period of about three weeks. Curiously, tapering off the smoking behaviour may cause more severe craving for nicotine than suddenly stopping (*cold turkey*).

There are many who are not easily convinced of the powerful addictive properties of nicotine. They should take to heart what happened during a tobacco workers' strike in Italy at the end of 1992. Cigarette supplies were interrupted for more than 30 days, emptying the shelves in tobacco stores. Those deprived of the drug smoked whatever they could get hold of, from cigars to aromatic herbs, and crossed national borders to buy smoking materials. The black market boomed and prices rose by 10%. Personal conversations became obsessed with the problem, and increased nervousness and irritability led some addicts to snatch lighted cigarettes from the lips of passers-by in the street.

In marijuana, the main active psychotropic principle is delta-9-tetrahydrocannabinol or THC. Some tolerance to this drug does develop, and is associated with a cross-tolerance to alcohol, but whether there is a real withdrawal syndrome is still a matter for debate. Although THC produces fewer physiological and psychological effects than most other drugs of abuse, including alcohol and nicotine, the fact that it does affect the CNS has been regarded as a matter for concern. However, there is said to be little evidence that any of these toxic effects is irreversible, though some observers claim that chronic use may lead ultimately to mental deterioration, apathy and general loss of ambition. It should be remembered, of course, that marijuana is a plant product and is usually smoked; it should not be surprising, therefore, to learn that chronic smoking of the drug can produce adverse effects on the respiratory system, including possible lung cancer. The question as to whether it is logical to ban marijuana, in view of its relatively low toxicity, when drugs like tobacco and alcohol are freely permitted, will be raised again in Chap. 31 (p. 222).

30

Addiction: Is There a Cure?

To cease smoking is the easiest thing I ever did.
I ought to know because I've done it a thousand times.

Mark Twain (1835–1910)

Cocaine isn't habit forming. I should know —
I've been using it for years.

Tallulah Bankhead (1903–68)

Ever since severe drug addiction has been regarded as an *illness*, the medical profession has explored many ways to effect a permanent cure. As Mark Twain implied, although temporary remission is not too difficult to bring about, relapse is frequently the discouraging long-term outcome. It is true that some addicts show spontaneous and total cure over the years, e.g., about 10–15% of opiate users stop taking the drug voluntarily in their thirties and forties. However, this still leaves us with a high proportion of inveterate, hard-core addicts.

To stop taking the addictive agent for good is, of course, the only genuine cure, but the motivation to achieve this must arise from the patient himself as a result of psychological and social readjustments. In the early years of the last century, the development of various schools of psychotherapy led to the hope that their approach would make it possible to reveal, and remove, the underlying psychological roots of drug abuse. Results, however, were disappointing. In 1958, the pooled records of 30 New York psychoanalysts indicated that they enjoyed a 14% remission rate, a figure not significantly different from the spontaneous one. This seems hardly surprising. After all, if the psychoanalytical treatment of psychosis, almost certainly the outcome of genetically-based neurotransmitter imbalance, is ineffective, then there is little reason to expect that psychoanalysis would successfully cure drug-induced neurotransmitter imbalance. If we further postulate that the potential drug addict has some neurotransmitter abnormality in the first place, making the recourse to psychotropic agents particularly rewarding, then the failure of psychoanalytical therapy becomes even more understandable.

Quite a different matter is the provision of psychological support and rehabilitation once the highly motivated addict has been restored temporarily to a drug-free environment and way of life. The fact that self-help organizations like Alcoholics Anonymous (AA), Narcotics Anonymous and many others are so well-known is a tribute to their undoubted success. And even if adjuvant drugs are used to encourage the patient in some way or other to forswear the abuse of psychotropic substances, reinforcement by physical and psychological rehabilitation programmes is essential if relapse is to be avoided.

However, we shall confine ourselves here to the various ways in which other drugs can be employed to help the addict, either by discouraging him from taking the addictive agent in the first place, or by relieving the symptoms of withdrawal once he decides to give it up, or by providing him with some relatively harmless substitute drug on a long-term basis. But before considering examples of these strategies, we must admit that using drugs to prevent or alleviate the adverse effects of abusing other drugs makes no great sense. It leads to no real cure, and the adjuvant drugs have their own toxicities and side effects. The truth is that the illness (if such it is) of compulsive self-administration of psychotropic substances is more than just a pharmacological problem, though the drugs in question do, of course, have pharmacological actions on the central nervous system.

There are, unfortunately, relatively few drugs which can effectively discourage the abuse of addictive agents. One ingenious way would be to interfere with the metabolism of these agents in the body in such a way that an abnormal metabolite, or a normal one at unusually high levels, is produced, causing intolerably unpleasant symptoms for the patient. The only real example of this approach is the use of disulfiram (Antabuse) in the treatment of alcoholism.[1] Ethyl alcohol is metabolized to acetic acid via an intermediate substance, acetaldeyhde. The acetaldehyde does not normally accumulate in the body because it is rapidly converted to acetic acid by the enzyme aldehyde dehydrogenase. Disulfiram inhibits this enzyme so that the acetaldehyde levels build up and cause disagreeable effects. Fifteen minutes after an alcoholic on disulfiram takes an alcohol-containing drink, his face becomes beet red and he experiences palpitations, chest pain, difficulty in breathing (dyspnoea), nausea and vomiting. The whole process is, in effect, a kind of pharmacological aversion therapy, making the addict most reluctant to indulge his craving for a drink.

By itself, disulfiram is relatively non-toxic and has few side effects, e. g., tiredness, dizziness, skin rashes, and gastro-intestinal discomfort, and these tend to disappear after one or two weeks if administration of the drug is continued. The success of disulfiram treatment depends on having a highly motivated patient with a stable lifestyle who is prepared to combine the therapy with appropriate counselling and rehabilitation. At one time Alcoholics Anonymous disapproved of using the drug as a crutch in treatment, but most groups today accept its value.

A drug of this kind is not known for the opioids, but the existence of the so-called partial agonists (see Chap. 13, p. 93) makes a rather similar approach at least theoretically possible. If given beforehand, the partial agonist, by occupying the morphine receptors in the brain, should block the euphoric and other central actions of the opioids, and so discourage the addict from resorting to the more potent agonists. A wide range of partial agonists is now available, from those like naloxone and naltrexone (which are virtually 100% antagonists) to pentazocine (Talwin) and buprenorphine (Buprenex) which have considerable agonist activity, and have been successfully used as analgesics with reduced *abuse potential*. Unfortunately, the pure antagonists naloxone and naltrexone have turned out to be rather unsatisfactory for discouraging the abuse of morphine and heroin. Naltrexone has the longer half-life (about 24 hours), so needs to be given orally only once a day, and it is relatively free of side effects. However, after about 30 to 60 days most potential addicts refuse to continue taking the drug because of vague unpleasant effects such as loss of energy.

Although buprenorphine is actually about 25 to 50 times more potent than morpine as an analgesic, and possesses a longer duration of action, its withdrawal symptoms are said not to be very severe. This is presumably because of its antagonist properties. However, like nalorphine (see Chap. 28, p. 199), it has some unpleasant psychotomimetic activity. Its use as a partial agonist to block the *"high"* induced by morphine and heroin is, therefore, disappointing. The more successful use of buprenorphine is as a substitute for methadone in methadone maintenance therapy (see later).

An already addicted subject who wishes to *kick the habit* will, of course, suffer the agonies of the withdrawal syndrome if he follows the *cold turkey* route to complete abstinence. Not only that, the abrupt cessation of certain addictive drugs, especially barbiturates or alcohol, may be fatal. On the assumption that withdrawal symptoms are related to abnormal brain levels of neurotransmitters, a specific approach to relieving the withdrawal syndrome would be to give a drug or drugs which could restore the transmitter levels to normal by antagonistic or other actions. This has so far been little explored, mainly because we are still ignorant about which neurotransmitters are involved in drug addiction. It is more usual to mitigate the very unpleasant symptoms of withdrawal by administering an analogue with similar, but milder, actions, or some other drugs which can relieve these symptoms by non-specific mechanisms.

With opiates, for example, the drug commonly used to cover withdrawal is the synthetic morphine analogue methadone. Methadone is preferred here for a number of reasons. It is effective by mouth, and since it is longer acting than morphine or heroin, it need not be given more frequently than once or twice a day. Its longer half life ($t_{1/2}$) also means that, although it does induce physical dependence, the withdrawal symptoms are far less distressing than those produced by the more potent opiates; they are, however, more protracted. Once the methadone has replaced the morphine or heroin in the body, the methadone itself can then be tailed off with much less discomfort for the addict. Finally, he or she is drug-free and ready for rehabilitation.

Barbiturate withdrawal can be covered with oral pentobarbitone, which is given to establish a stabilizing level for one to two days and then gradually and patiently reduced in dosage over a period of ten days to three weeks. Some physicians prefer to use the long-acting phenobarbitone which is more effective in suppressing convulsions.

Ethyl alcohol withdrawal presents somewhat different problems. There is no suitable analogue that could be used as cover, and one has to suppress the hyperexcitability with various types of depressant, e.g., barbiturates and other sedatives, anti-convulsants or anxiolytic agents such as diazepam (Valium). Almost as important with alcoholics is the need to correct the malnutrition and vitamin deficiencies which they almost invariably show (they do not eat a healthy mixed diet but depend on the alcohol for their calorie intake), and to treat any liver damage.

To wean cigarette smokers from their unhealthy addiction implies, in effect, curing their dependence on nicotine. It might be thought ingenious to provide them cigarettes with a lower nicotine content, but this backfires by encouraging them to smoke more often and to puff (and so inhale) more vigorously. These adjustments allow them to maintain the plasma nicotine at addictive levels, and, moreover, to increase the health hazards of smoking (e.g., from increased intake of carbon monoxide and other toxic products of combustion).

A better approach is to stop smoking altogether, and administer the pure addictive agent in the form of nicotine gums or skin patches. Nicotine gum is chewed, releasing the active substance which is then absorbed through the oral mucosa. But there are some problems: the amount of nicotine released depends on the vigour of chewing, and the dosage may, therefore, be too small or too large. Since nicotine is a basic substance, its absorption varies with the pH of the saliva; and if some rather acid liquids have been ingested beforehand (e.g., coffee, soda), the consequently increased ionization of the nicotine will depress its mucosal absorption.

Nicotine-containing skin patches, attached to the upper arm or torso and replaced after 24 hours, provide more reliable absorption over a longer period of time. The nicotine content of the patches is reduced gradually over six weeks to several months, at which time it is hoped that the craving for cigarettes will have been eliminated. However, long-term results of this treatment are discouraging; only about 15% of subjects manage to give up smoking for a full year afterwards. As already mentioned, such drug therapy must be accompanied by behavioural counselling and psychological support. Nicotine patches are not free of side effects. Some subjects experience insomnia or nightmares if the patch is not removed overnight. Attempts to *cheat*, by seeking the additional comfort of a smoke, may lead to the absorption of too much nicotine, and this can be dangerous for those at risk of a heart attack.

The use of a substitute drug, rather than aiming for the drug-free state, has been applied particularly to the treatment of opiate addiction. The idea of *curing* addiction to one drug by giving another similar agent with similar addictive properties would, as suggested above, seem rather defeatist. But Drs. V.P. Dole and Marie Nyswander (Mrs. Dole) boldly introduced this controversial concept in 1965, as a reaction to the failure of psychotherapy and the severe relapse rate in narcotic addicts treated by total withdrawal.[2] Dole and Nyswander felt that many opiate addicts had some profound central nervous system abnormality, perhaps biochemical in nature, which made the relief provided by narcotic analgesics absolutely necessary for a reasonably happy existence. Complete withdrawal was, therefore, regarded as a hopeless goal, and these unfortunate people had to be given some sort of drug treatment throughout life. Dole and Nyswander chose oral methadone, and their regime is known as *methadone maintenance therapy* (MMT).

Undoubtedly, methadone has many advantages over morphine or heroin if you have to be dependent on opiates. Its effectiveness taken by mouth in orange juice, its longer duration of action and the milder nature of its withdrawal syndrome have already been mentioned. Dole and Nyswander also claimed that, although the subjects receiving methadone did not experience the euphoric "*high*" of morphine or heroin, they were not tempted to take those drugs in addition to the methadone. This was because the methadone effectively blocked the euphoria normally induced by the stronger opiates. The social effects of MMT are also beneficial. The addict is provided at special clinics with free daily doses of methadone under controlled conditions, and does not have to buy street heroin from pushers at ruinous costs. Oral administration obviates the dangers of intravenous self-infection (dirty syringes, skin infections, hepatitis, AIDS, etc.). The improvement in health and morale allows the addict to take up gainful employment, and to escape from the clutches of the criminal underworld.[3]

However, it is now generally believed that Dole and Nyswander painted rather too rosy a picture of MMT. Methadone does not completely block opiate euphoria, but merely increases the dose required to produce a "*high*". Addicts are grateful for methadone handouts when street prices of heroin become exorbitant, but they find the substitute less than satisfying. They tend to cheat by taking other drugs to *top up*, e.g., heroin, barbiturates or amphetamines; and are liable to revert to street drugs when prices fall. Addicts maintained on methadone are far from normal; they show many of the long-term effects of chronic opiate administration, e.g., constipation, constricted pupils, insomnia, impotence and excessive sweating. Another possible danger of MMT is that methadone may find its way out of the special clinics and into the hands of the pushers. Buprenorphine has been advocated as a useful alternative to methadone in MMT, and, in some addicts, administration every 48 hours may be sufficient.

It is obviously difficult, even impossible, to discourage the widespread use of *recreational* drugs, and to wean users off them once they have become addicted. Many societies, therefore, have tried to eliminate or reduce the availability of addictive drugs by social, legal and punitive measures at the government level. This has not been a striking success, either, and there is an increasing trend today to experiment with more permissive, less draconian and less costly policies. These strategies will not, of course, eradicate drug abuse, but might lead to a diminished involvement of the criminal underworld. The next chapter will consider some of these possibilities, which have been summarized under the general heading of *harm reduction*.

31

Harm Reduction: The Middle Way

That humanity at large will ever be able to dispense
with Artificial Paradises seems very unlikely. Most
men and women lead lives at the worst so painful, at
the best so monotonous, poor and limited that the urge
to escape, the longing to transcend themselves if only
for a few moments, is and always has been one of the
principal appetites of the soul.

Aldous Huxley, *The Doors of Perception* (1954)

About 30 years ago, staid readers of the London *Times* were scandalized to
come across a full-page advertisement advocating a substantial
liberalization of the laws concerning the possession and use of cannabis
(marijuana). One of the signatories was a well-known British psychiatrist
who, at the time, enjoyed considerable popularity as a television
personality (Sir David Stafford-Clark).

Perhaps as a result of this publicity, a Sub-Committee on Cannabis was
set up by the UK Advisory Committee on Drug Dependence under the
chairmanship of Barbara Wootton. This committee produced its
controversial report in 1968. Its members were disturbed by the severity of
the penalties then inflicted for possession of cannabis and they deprecated
in particular the frequent imposition of prison sentences (often on first
offenders) for being found with quite small quantities. They recommended
a substantial reduction in the sentences permitted by law for the
possession, sale or supply of the drug.

The main recommendations of the Wootton Report were
unequivocally rejected by the government of the time, and the committee

members came under intensive criticism from certain quarters, who complained that they had advocated the complete legalization of cannabis. This was not true. Their Report stated: "In the interests of public health it is necessary to maintain restrictions on the availability and use of the drug ... there is no alternative to the criminal law and its penalties."

Demands for relaxation of severe legal penalties for possessing and using cannabis have continued to surface from time to time in the UK, USA and elsewhere, provoked to some extent by the publication of much new material on the pharmacology of cannabis. This would seem to show that the use and abuse of this drug is relatively harmless, and certainly less deleterious than indulgence in socially acceptable agents such as alcohol and tobacco (see Chap. 29, p. 210). Many experts, however, would claim, even today, that our knowledge about the short-term and long-term effects of cannabis administration remains incomplete because, in the words of the Wootton Report, the findings "do not all point in the same direction". Cannabis is a tricky drug to investigate, and there is considerable scope for disagreement over the interpretation of the experimental results. This is partly due to the chemical properties of the active principles, and to the rather ill-defined and unspectacular range of physiological and pharmacological actions which they produce.

The plant was given the botanical name *Cannabis sativa* by Linnaeus in 1753, but it had been known to mankind for thousands of years. It grows wild in the Americas, Africa and Asia, and can be successfully cultivated in any reasonably warm climate. It is a commercial source of hemp fibre, and the seeds are used for extraction of an oil and for feeding caged birds. The medicinal application of cannabis as a *narcotic* may have originated in China, but by the Christian era the plant had spread to India, Persia and the Middle East. It reached Europe around the sixteenth century.

The two main preparations of cannabis are marijuana and hashish, the latter being the more potent because it is derived from the resin scraped off the female plant (deadlier than the male!). Marijuana (known familiarly as grass, pot or weed) consists of the crushed leaves and flowers, and is rolled into cigarettes (reefers). Hashish (hash) is often smoked in a pipe, but may be incorporated in an ordinary hand-rolled cigarette made with tobacco. Nowadays, a concentrated alcoholic extract of cannabis containing the most important active principle tetrahydrocannabinol (THC), isolated in pure form only since 1970, is available. This may be dribbled onto an ordinary cigarette and allowed to dry before smoking.

In the East, there is a longer tradition of cannabis as a recreational drug, and methods of taking it are more varied and sophisticated. It may be incorporated into a confection with butter, sugar and flour, or made into an intoxicating drink. If smoked, a water pipe is used to ensure that tars and other irritating water-soluble substances are removed from the smoke without losing the active water-insoluble THC. This is wise, as it has now been discovered that smoking cannabis is just as likely to cause lung cancer as smoking tobacco, a fact which should have surprised no one. The combustion of the dried leaves of *any* plant would be expected to produce roughly the same kind of lethal mixture of tars and carbon monoxide.[1] In fact, recent research has indicated that cannabis smoking may generate 55% more tar than a harsh tobacco leaf. Moreover, it is the customary ritual to draw the smoke from cannabis deeply into the lungs and retain it there as long as possible. Against this, it must be admitted that cannabis smokers do not take more than two to six reefers a day, compared with the 20 to 60 per day for the heavy smoker.

The chemical make-up of cannabis resin is extremely complex. The most important components are the oily cannabinoids, of which THC is the most active. The amounts and proportions of these cannabinoids vary according to the source of the plant, and furthermore the THC content tends to decrease as the sample ages. This explains to some extent the conflicting reports that have been published on the central and other actions of cannabis.

Cannabinoids are very fat-soluble substances which undergo metabolism in the body to scores of metabolites. Some of these are also psychoactive. For this reason, all these substances tend to cumulate and persist in the fatty tissues for a considerable time (rather like DDT). This provides a marked contrast with alcohol, which is totally eliminated from the body in a relatively short time, and whose metabolites are simple compounds readily dealt with by the organism. The long-term effects of the many metabolites of cannabis have still not been fully documented.

The subjective effects of smoking cannabis show a rapid onset, owing to the high solubility of the active agents. At low doses, the smoker feels something akin to alcoholic intoxication, with an elevated mood and increased self-confidence. There is euphoria with bouts of senseless giggling, a loss of tension and inhibitions and a desire to remain undisturbed in a state of contemplation. There are distortions of space and time; in particular, time is experienced as longer than clock time, or may dissolve into an alarming feeling of timelessness. Recent memory, learning and selective attention are affected, and the capacity to perform mental arithmetic and tests of coordination is definitely impaired.

High dosage and habitual use may lead to psychosis-like episodes which normally disappear on stopping the drug. So-called *mini-delusions* are liable to occur. These are false beliefs which, however, do not have the overwhelmingly distressing effects of true psychotic delusions. For example, one subject complained that whenever she bathed after smoking marijuana, she believed that there was a man in the bath beside her. Although this aroused feelings of excitement and anxiety, she never looked to see if the man was really there. Chronic use produces some degree of tolerance, and psychological dependence develops rapidly. Physical dependence, however, is not thought to occur. Individuals who become psychologically dependent are said to lose interest in the outside world, and passively give themselves over to lethargy and daydreaming. This state is rather pretentiously described as the *amotivational syndrome.*

It is not well-known that marijuana also has therapeutic applications, some of them going back many centuries, e.g., for the treatment of pain and inflammation. Even today, THC (marketed as dronabinol or Marinol) has its advocates for suppressing the nausea often caused by cancer chemotherapy, for lowering the increased intra-ocular pressure of glaucoma, and for relieving the painful muscular spasms seen in multiple sclerosis (MS) and after spinal injuries. These uses have been generally opposed by the medical profession because of the psychoactive properties of the drug, but in the UK treatment with cannabis was licensed in 2000. Nonetheless, there are safer, more acceptable, drugs available to treat the above conditions. The recent discovery of peripheral THC receptors in the body does open up the possibility of devising synthetic THC analogues that might act selectively on those peripheral sites, but not on the central nervous system.

The pharmacology of cannabis has been dealt with in some depth here[2] because it illustrates rather well some of the dilemmas that bedevil society's efforts to eradicate the problem of drug addiction. It is obviously irrational to regard cannabis as any more dangerous than tobacco, and a good case could be made for rating it actually safer than alcohol. Clearly, there are reasonable arguments for legalizing the drug. The question is: Do we need to add yet another addictive agent to those already accepted by society, especially when we know that a certain proportion of the subjects who experiment with these so-called soft drugs will eventually escalate to hard drugs like heroin or cocaine?

On the other hand, a Savonarola (the moralistic Florentine reformer, 1452–98) would no doubt prefer to stand the arguments on their heads, and use pharmacological facts to support a total ban of tobacco, alcohol *and* cannabis. But such measures would inevitably provoke a violent counter-reaction, and the history of prohibition in the USA in the 1920s is an object lesson in this respect. Even the widely publicized and costly wars initiated by the USA and other industrialized countries against hard drugs have not been conspicuously successful. The opposite extreme — to legalize *all* drugs of addiction — would certainly undercut the profits for the international drug cartels and the pushers, but would surely be a policy of despair, and of possible disaster for our urban communities. What happened in Zurich in 1988 provided a spectacular example of these dangers. Officials in the Swiss capital designated a park in which drugs could be sold and used without interference. A few years later, the experiment had to be terminated after the park became a haven for dealers, prostitutes and addicts from all over Europe. More successful was the legalization of cannabis cafes in Holland, leading, it was said, to an actual decrease in the abuse of the drug.

In view of the fact that many psychoactive drugs have been known, and used, for thousands of years, why, in the twenty-first century, do we find ourselves on the horns of so desperate a dilemma?

Undoubtedly one important factor is the loss of powerful informal controls operating within traditional rural societies. For example, alcohol-drinking behaviour in a typical African village is still controlled by cultural habits and taboos in a community tightly knit by family bonds, and where everyone knows everyone else. When the villagers leave for the big city searching for a better life, they often end up in urban slums, and the problem of alcoholism explodes. Similar controls exist among the opium-growing hill tribes of Northern Thailand, and in Central and South American cultures that use potent hallucinogens for ritual purposes.[3]

Virginia Berridge and Griffith Edwards, in their book, *Opium and the People*,[4] have studied in detail the popular use of drugs like morphine, cannabis and cocaine in early Victorian England. The importation of foreign opium (mainly from Turkey) was completely unrestricted until 1868, and small-scale attempts were even made to cultivate it domestically in the early nineteenth century. One area of England, where the use of opium and various preparations of opium, e.g., laudanum, was particularly widespread, was the Fen District, with its impoverished rural population. This covers parts of East Anglia (Lincolnshire, Cambridgeshire,

Huntingdonshire and Norfolk) and was at that time a remote, low-lying and marshy region with few medical practitioners, and a working population prone to ague, painful rheumatism and neuralgia.

Opium and its preparations were not generally prescribed by doctors, but were bought quite freely in druggists and small grocery stores. In Charles Kingsley's novel *Alton Locke*, a character remarks: "Yow goo [You go] into druggist's shop o' market day, into Cambridge, and you'll see the little boxes, doozens and doozens, a'ready on the counter; and never a ven-man's [fen-man's] wife goo by, but what calls in for her pennord [pennyworth] o'elevation to last her out the week ... Well, it keeps women folk quiet, it do; and it's mortal good agin ago [ague] pains."[5]

Berridge and Edwards comment: "It [i.e., regular and widespread opium use in the Fens] had been, in its time, a notable example of the operation of a system of open availability ... It had demonstrated how a population could succeed in controlling by informed social mechanisms its consumption of the drug, with only minimal medicinal and legislative intervention."

Be that as it may, morphine possessed the same properties of toxicity, tolerance and addiction in the nineteenth century as it does today. The use of opium preparations in the Fens, though perhaps not out of control, must have caused much morbidity and mortality among the rural population. The *doping* of young babies was widespread, and there was a variety of special mixtures with suggestive names available for this purpose: Godfrey's Cordial, Atkinson's Infant Preservative, Street's Infant Quietness and many others. Not surprisingly, infant mortality rates in Fenland towns were extremely high, and possibly some of these deaths were premeditated. Among adults, deaths were recorded from accidental overdosage as a result of ill-trained pharmacists providing the wrong dose or mixing up different preparations. Such tragedies attracted little attention unless the victims came from the upper echelons of society, and the medical profession, such as it was at that time, was rarely called in.

Nevertheless, concern about drug usage began to grow among the authorities from about 1830 onwards, and during the following decades provoked something of a localized *war on drugs*. However, as Berridge and Edwards wisely observe: "Concentration on simple statistical results without an awareness of social context or economic reality produced a situation which justified the restriction of open sale of the drug. Opium, as elsewhere, was the scapegoat for broader defects in the society of the time."

(Is there not, perhaps, a lesson here for those who, today, wage their costly *wars on drugs*, but now on a bitter global scale?)

A number of factors operating over the past 150 years or so have greatly exacerbated the problem of drug abuse in Western societies. The Industrial Revolution and the consequent movement of rural populations to the growing cities bred an urban proletariat, and led to the breakdown of family and cultural bonds. Class tensions in these cities encouraged a belief that urban opium use was more threatening to the structure of society than opium use in the countryside. The situation deteriorated during the twentieth century as a result of the availability of other addictive drugs, and the improvement of global communications, which allowed such drugs to be readily transported from their countries of origin. US cities appear to have suffered more from these changes, perhaps because poverty and urban decay were compounded there by ethnic and racial antagonisms and well-entrenched criminal organizations like the Mafia.

Certain technical advances have also played an important role, e.g., the chemical isolation of the pure active principles and the consequent feasibility of injecting them by syringe. An intravenous injection leads to immediate high blood levels of a drug and faster penetration into the central nervous system. It is now realized that the rapid onset (and cessation) of the central actions of many addictive drugs leads to extreme euphoria (*the rush*), followed shortly afterwards by a *crash*. This results in immediate conditioning and the rapid establishment of dependency. This did not happen when opium and its preparations were available only in oral forms, which no doubt explains why serious addiction rarely surfaced as a problem in the Fens.

More controversial is the influence of the medical profession in alerting the public to the dangers of drug abuse, largely by *medicalizing* it as a disease requiring treatment. It is often forgotten that doctors were not always highly regarded, and that their earnings in the middle 1800s were only in the upper blue collar range! All that changed with improvement in medical education (stimulated in the USA, for example, by the 1910 Flexner Report) and the formation of professional organizations like the American Medical Association and the General Medical Council in Great Britain. Pharmacists also enhanced their status for similar reasons. By 1925, doctors came third in social prestige, following bankers and college professors, and after 1933 won, and retained, top place with earnings to match. The increasing influence of the medical establishment within society and on government policies led to stiffer legal controls, e.g., a series of *Dangerous Drugs* Acts in the UK from 1920 onwards, which restricted the prescribing of such drugs (especially the active principles) to authorized professionals. This encouraged criminal elements to play a more active part in obtaining supplies of addictive drugs for illegal *recreational* use.

All these various factors, and perhaps many others, have contributed to the unprecedented crisis that we face today. But if attempts to eradicate drug abuse by throwing larger and larger sums of money into law enforcement policies have proved a costly failure, and if the outright legalization of all drugs of addiction would be, to say the least, a dangerous gamble, what other options do we have? In the past few years, many drug specialists both here and abroad have begun to advocate a "Middle Way" known as *grudging toleration* or (more commonly) *harm reduction*. The idea behind harm reduction is that addiction should be seen, at worst, as a disease requiring treatment, and not as an absolute evil to be extirpated at any cost.

Professor Arnold S. Trebach, President of the Drug Policy Foundation in Washington D.C., explains: "The essence [of harm reduction] is the acceptance of the enduring reality of drug use, the absurdity of even attempting to create a drug-free society and the need to treat drug users and abusers as basically decent human beings." Support for this approach is said to be growing internationally. In Europe, many cities and provinces have signed the Frankfurt Resolution, which calls for easing prohibitions on marijuana, free availability of clean syringe needles and treatment for all who seek it. A conference held in Washington D.C. in May 1993, attended by drug specialists, law enforcement officers, judges, physicians and social scientists, also favoured in general a moderate programme of harm reduction, though no agreement in detail on exactly how to achieve this goal was reached at that meeting.

ENVOI

Was Aldous Huxley right? History teaches us that the most far-reaching social reforms and revolutions have so far failed dismally to establish an earthly Utopia where mankind is freed from pain, misery and monotony. It is not surprising that some may feel that all that is left for us are the Artificial Paradises induced by psychoactive chemicals. Yet these potent agents are themselves capable of producing their own brand of pain and misery, even death.

We have learned that psychoactive drugs act on the brain to modify thought, feeling and mood because that organ is regulated by chemical substances (neurotransmitters, neuroinhibitors and neuroregulators). Does this mean that there are certain flaws or defects in the neuroregulatory chemistry of the human brain that are primarily responsible for our pain and misery, and that no amount of tinkering with the organization of society itself can ever compensate for these flaws? In other words, is brain chemistry stronger than politics? As our knowledge of the brain grows, we *may* be able to pin-point the sites of these neuroregulatory defects (if they really exist), and perhaps then discover a drug that can selectively neutralize them without causing dependence or other unwanted effects. I doubt that such a drug exits, or could ever exist, in spite of all the recent dangerous ballyhoo over the selective serotonin (5-HT) re-uptake inhibitor fluoxetine (Prozac).[6]

Unfortunately, there may, in fact, be something fundamentally addictive about normal brain function, for even the higher animals are not immune to the lure of psychoactive drugs. This may not be due to any real flaw, but is simply the inevitable result of the need, during evolution, to develop a mechanism for avoiding the painful and harmful, and for seeking out the pleasurable and harmless in the environment. This principle of pain-avoidance and pleasure-seeking must act through memory and learning, and obviously has considerable survival value for the organism.

Recent research suggests that there is a neural mechanism called long-term potentiation (LTP) which is crucial in the laying down of memory and learning. LTP occurs when repeated impulses crossing a synapse linking two neurones result in a positive feedback, which facilitates further synaptic transmission. Similar synaptic facilitation or reinforcement mechanisms could well play an important role during the conditioning effects of doses of a pleasure-producing drug, and be responsible for the development of physical dependence (cf. p. 189). If so, a propensity to habituation and addiction (and not necessarily only to drugs) may be an inescapable neural property of our brains, which are, after all, not exempt from the pressures of Darwinian selection.

As we have emphasized throughout this book, drugs that are able to cure or alleviate disease will continue to play a necessary and important role in medical treatment. However, in the course of time, a greater stress on preventive medicine, and the increasing use of gene therapy in the treatment of heritable disease, may well diminish the need for medication with chemical substances, though this is unlikely ever to vanish completely. Drugs that can usefully alter sensation, e.g., narcotics, anxiolytics, hypnotics, anaesthetics, will remain of value, even though many of them may cause varying degrees of physical dependence. Drugs that are used purely for recreational purposes, but have no genuine therapeutic applications, would ideally be expunged from our pharmacopoeias. We also must not forget to pay more attention to the serious dangers posed by the industrial chemicals released into our air, water, soil and food. As Paracelsus so presciently observed some 500 years ago: Nothing is without poison ...

Notes and References

Introduction

1. See Paul Davies, *Superforce: The Search for a Grand Unified Theory of Nature* (London: Heinemann, 1984), pp. 162, 238, 242–43, for a sympathetic exposition of this theory. However, Murray Gell-Mann in *The Quark and the Jaguar: Adventures in the Simple and the Complex* (New York: W.H. Freeman and Co., 1994), pp. 212–13, regards the concept "so ridiculous as to merit no further discussion".

2. For an account of recent theories of the origins of life on earth, see Noam Laha, *Biogenesis: Theories of Life's Origin* (Oxford: Oxford University Press, 1999). An article by Robert M. Hazen in *Scientific American*, Vol. 284, No. 4, April 2001, pp. 76–85, suggests that minerals present in the earth's crust may have played an important catalytic role in converting simple carbon compounds (CO, CO_2, CH_4) to the more complex molecules required for life.

3. Albert Szent-Györgyi's views on the early development of life on earth can be found in *The Living State: With Observations on Cancer* (New York & London: Academic Press, 1972), pp. 48–49, 56; and *The Living State and Cancer* (New York & Basel: Marcel Dekker, Inc., 1978), p.17.

4. A pamphlet outlining the chemistry of biological free radicals and their possible involvement in tissue injury (e.g., emphysema; the toxicities of radiation, air pollution and carbon tetrachloride; and the aging process) was published by Upjohn Company, Kalamazoo, Michigan in 1985: Joseph C. Fantone and Peter A. Ward, *Oxygen-Derived Radicals and Their Metabolites: Relationship to Tissue Injury*. For a more detailed account, see J. Feher, G. Cosmós and A. Vereckei, *Free Radical Reactions in Medicine* (Berlin, Heidelberg, New York: Springer Verlag, 1985).

5. Brian Inglis, *A History of Medicine* (Cleveland: World Publishing Co., 1965), p. 7. The full quotation reads as follows: "The medicine man did not — and to this day does not — usually practise medicine in the ordinary sense. He practised magic, with healing his objective — though, as the assumption was that disease was caused by magic, or witchcraft, the remedy was often actually designed to harm, or kill off, or frighten off, the purveyors — man or evil spirits — in the hope that this would allow their victim to recover."

6. Some implications of the completion of the Human Genome Project (HGP) for the future of scientific medicine have been discussed in recent issues of the *British Medical Journal* (*BMJ*) and *Scientific American*. The *BMJ* explains the medical aspects of genetic testing, eugenics and pharmacogenomics. *Scientific American* covers much the same ground, but goes into more scientific detail. *Gene Therapy*, published first in September 1995, outlines the aim and

problems of this new approach to therapeutics. See "The Impact of New Technologies in Medicine: The Human Genome Project", *British Medical Journal*, No. 7220 (13 November 1999), pp. 1282–86; "The Business of the Human Genome", *Scientific American*, Vol. 283, No. 1 (July 2000), pp. 48–69; "Revolutions in Science", *Scientific American*, Special Issue (2000), pp. 52–55.

7. See "Drug Giant Calls for Genetic Screening". *Guardian Weekly*, Vol. 162, No. 17 (20–26 April 2000), p. 7.

Chapter 1

1. This account of George Washington's final illness is taken from Barbara Griggs, *Green Pharmacy: A History of Herbal Medicine* (London, Jill Norman & Hobhouse, 1981), pp. 154–55.

2. See Martin Kaufman, *Homeopathy in America* (Baltimore: Johns Hopkins University Press, 1971).

3. See Robert Blake, *Disraeli* (New York: St. Martin's Press, 1967), pp. 632–33, 747.

4. *Nature*, Vol. 333 (30 June 1988), p. 816.

5. "Randomized controlled trial of homeopathy versus placebo in perennial allergic rhinitis, with overview of four trial series", *British Medical Journal*, No. 7259 (19–26 August 2000), pp. 471–76.

6. More up-to-date and reliable figures are difficult to obtain. The Public Citizens Foundation, a consumer advocate organization in Washington, DC, claimed recently (2001) that "every year approximately 100,000 Americans are killed by adverse drug reactions, while another 1.5 million are injured so severely that they need to be hospitalized."

7. Linus Pauling, *How to Live Longer* (New York, Freeman & Co., 1986), Chap. 11, p. 95. The expression "toximolecular medicine" was coined in 1979 by Bernard Riland.

8. Joel G. Hardman and Lee E. Limbird (eds.), *Goodman and Gilman's The Pharmacological Basis of Therapeutics*, 10th ed. (New York: McGraw-Hill, 2001), pp. 1750, 1760. The tenth edition of this authoritative work appeared during preparation of the present text and will be referred to as hereafter as *Goodman and Gilman*.

9. Professor S. Feldman, "Personal Communication".

Chapter 2

1. Other technological developments which have enormously accelerated the output of new synthetic compounds in recent years are *combinatory chemistry*, and the increased precision of separative and purification processes. In

combinatory chemistry, synthesis is carried out on a solid support system, and literally thousands of new molecules (e.g., peptides) can be made by a single chemist in a single week. In this way, drug firms can speed up the discovery of new drugs, though still in a rather hit-or-miss way. See "A Revolution in Drug Discovery", *British Medical Journal*, No. 7261 (9 September 2000), pp. 581–82.

2. Professor S. Feldman, Personal Communication.

Chapter 3

1. D.R. Laurence and P.N. Bennett, *Clinical Pharmacology* (Edinburgh, London and New York: Churchill Livingstone, 1980). This book has long been an invaluable source of information about drugs and their use in therapeutics, and manages also to be extremely well-written, often entertaining and refreshingly anecdotal. Regretfully, since the fifth edition published in 1980, no later revision has appeared. The statistics quoted here are, however, somewhat bizarrely expressed. For example, the British figures really mean that doctors held a sufficient number of consultations to provide, if evenly distributed, each member of the population with three apiece. But actually, since a lot of people do not consult a doctor, many patients were obviously seeing their doctor far more than three times a year. Moreover, these would receive far more than 1.6 prescription drugs per two consultations. The Australian figures also require a little thought.

2. Lynn Payer, *Medicine and Culture* (New York: Henry Holt & Co., 1988), pp. 23–25, 60–67, 73, 86–90. This hard-hitting medical journalist has also written *Disease-Mongers; How Doctors, Drug Companies and Insurers are Making You Feel Sick* (New York: John Wiley and Sons, Inc., 1993).

Chapter 4

1. *Journal of the American Medical Association (JAMA)*, Vol. 111 (1938), p. 919.

2. *JAMA*, Vol. 109 (1937), p. 1985; Vol. 111 (1938), p. 1567.

3. We owe the concepts of LD_{80}, ED_{50}, etc., to John William Trevan. See B. Holmstedt and G. Liljestrand (eds.), *Readings in Pharmacology* (New York: The Macmillan Co., 1963), Chap. VII, pp. 244–50.

4. Professor S. Feldman, Personal Communication.

5. "Foreword by Sir Andrew Huxley", in: W.D.M. Paton, *Man and Mouse: Animals in Medical Research* (Oxford: Oxford University Press, 1984), pp. v–vi.

6. W.D.M. Paton, *Man and Mouse: Animals in Medical Research* (Oxford: Oxford University Press, 1984), p. 160.

7. See Alan M. Goldberg and John M. Frazier, "Alternatives to Animals in Toxicity Testing", *Scientific American*, Vol. 261, No. 2 (1989), p. 24.

Chapter 5

1. This definition is taken from Bradford Hill, *Principles of Medical Statistics* (London: Hodder and Stoughton, 1977), and is quoted in D.R. Laurence and P. N. Bennett, *Clinical Pharmacology* (1980), Chap. 5, p. 70.
2. See Sidney M. Wolfe (ed.), *Worst Pills Best Pills*, Vol. 6, No. 5 (May 2000), pp. 33–34, a publication of the Public Citizen Health Research Group. See also: "UK Licence for Cisapride Suspended", *British Medical Journal*, No. 7256 (29 July 2000), p. 259.
3. The Public Citizen Research Group published in their *Health Letter*, Vol. 16, No. 5 (May 2000), p.4, an open letter to FDA Commissioner, Dr. Jane Henney, objecting to her decision to allow the withdrawn drug Propulsid to remain on pharmacy shelves for sale to the public until mid-August 2000. They conclude: "Unless the FDA forces Johnson and Johnson to promptly clear this drug off drug store shelves, a large number of further preventable deaths are certain to occur in the United States, mainly in people for whom there are numerous alternatives for the treatment of gastroesophageal reflux disease (GERD), also referred to as 'heartburn', the principal medical condition for which the drug is prescribed."

Chapter 6

1. This definition of an adverse or toxic reaction to a drug is paraphrased from D. R. Laurence and P.N. Bennett, *Clinical Pharmacology* (1980), Chap. 1, p. 8.
2. D.R. Laurence and P.N. Bennett, *Clinical Pharmacology* (1980), pp. 418–20.
3. The perplexing problems with practolol (Eraldin) are described fairly in D.R. Laurence and P.N. Bennett, *Clinical Pharmacology* (1980), pp. 18–20. Brian Inglis's approach in *The Diseases of Civilisation* (London: Hodder and Stoughton, 1981), pp. 13–15, is coloured by his obvious disillusionment with orthodox medicine in general.
4. For more about the dangers of triazolam (Halcion), see Chap. 27.
5. B.B. Brodie, "Physicochemical and Biochemical Aspects of Pharmacology" (The 1967 Albert Lasker Award Lecture), *JAMA*, Vol. 202, p. 600.
6. It was actually A. Motulsky in "Drug Reactions, Enzymes and Biochemical Genetics", *JAMA*, Vol. 165 (1957), pp. 835–37, who first suggested that idiosyncratic drug reactions might be caused by otherwise innocuous genetic traits and enzyme deficiencies. W. Kalow's book *Pharmacogenetics: Heredity and the Response to Drugs* was published by W.B. Saunders & Co. (Philadelphia, 1962). See the recent survey by W.W. Weber, *Pharmacogenetics* (New York: Oxford University Press, 1997).
7. W. Kalow and K. Genest. "A Method for the Detection of Atypical Forms of Serum Cholinesterase: Determination of Dibucaine Numbers", *Canadian Journal of Biochemistry*, Vol. 35 (1957), pp. 1305–17.

Chapter 7

1. *Goodman and Gilman* (2001), p. 1889, express the long half-life of DDT in the following striking way: "Elimination is estimated to occur at a rate of about 1% of stored DDT per day."
2. See *Worst Pills Best Pills*, Vol. 4, No. 5 (May 2000), pp. 39–40. The information is taken from the UK Committee on Safety of Medicines' warning to doctors, pharmacists, and the public, about a significant number of interactions between St. John's Wort and prescription drugs. The important point is made that "herbal supplements are not regulated as drugs ... and the amount of active ingredient can vary among preparations. Consequently, the degree of liver enzyme induction from different St. John's Wort preparations is also likely to vary."
3. See D.R. Laurence and P.N. Bennett, *Clinical Pharmacolog* (1980), Chap. 1, pp. 13–20.

Chapter 8

1. The most recent edition of *The Complete Drug Reference* (2001) lists 74 names for acetaminophen in the US and 33 in Canada.
2. *Physicians' Desk Reference (PDR)*, 53rd ed. (Montvale, NJ, USA: Medical Economics Co., Inc., 1999.)
3. This story is told by D.R. Laurence and P.N. Bennett in *Clinical Pharmacology* (1980), Chap. 7, p. 101.
4. Jeffrey K. Aronson, "Where name and image meet — The argument for adrenaline", *BMJ*, No. 7233 (19 February 2000), pp. 506–509.

Chapter 9

1. Brian Inglis, *Drugs, Doctors and Disease* (London: André Deutsch Ltd., 1965). Inglis's comments on the Kefauver Committee's findings are briefly recapitulated in his *The Diseases of Civilisation* (1981), pp. 133–35, 137.
2. Milton Silverman, Philip R. Lee and Mia Lydecker, *Prescriptions for Death: The Drugging of the Third World* (Berkeley, Los Angeles: University of California Press, 1982).
3. Brian Inglis, *The Diseases of Civilisation*, pp. 264–67.

Chapter 10

1. See p. 265. This quotation follows Brian Inglis's expressed opinion that "doctors are considered to have a low level of sales resistance — as, indeed, the low intellectual level of the drug advertisements in medical journals confirms."

2. A typical example of this is the response of the drug companies to the humanitarian disaster of widespread AIDS in Africa. The cost of the drugs needed to control this epidemic is far beyond the means of most of the governments involved, and certainly those of the individual patients. Governments that attempted to import the much cheaper generic drugs manufactured in, e.g., India, Thailand and Egypt, were threatened with law suits, on the grounds that patent rights were being infringed. The furore and anger aroused worldwide by this multinational callousness did, however, shame many firms to lower their prices, and withdraw their law suits (April 2001).
3. See Chap. 9, Note 1.
4. See Silverman, Lee and Lydecker, *Prescriptions for Death* (1982), pp. 137–38, and Tables 1–8.
5. Andrew Chetley, *A Healthy Business? World Health and the Pharmaceutical Industry* (London: Zed Books, 1990).

Chapter 11

1. For an up-to-date account of pharmacokinetics, see *Goodman and Gilman* (2001), Chap. 1, "The Dynamics of Drug Absorption, Distribution and Elimination", pp. 3–29.
2. Professor S. Feldman, Personal Communication.
3. An aerosol form of the semi-synthetic antidiuretic hormone (ADH) lypressin (Diapid) is also effective as a nasal spray, The nasal administration of insulin, given with adjuvants to improve absorption is promising, see *Goodman and Gilman* (2001), pp. 803 and 1701, for a review of recent attempts to find alternative routes of administration for these agents.

Chapter 12

1. For more about the blood-brain barrier, see *Goodman and Gilman* (2001), Chap. 1, p. 10 and Chap. 12, p. 297.

Chapter 13

1. For a detailed and up-to-date account of pharmacodynamics, see *Goodman and Gilman* (2001), Chap. 2, "Pharmacodynamics: Mechanisms of Drug Action and the Relationship between Drug Concentration and Effect", pp. 31–43. Laurence and Bennett, *Clinical Pharmacology* (1980) has a contribution (Chap. 3, p. 39) by J.W. Black on "How Drugs Act", written for a non-specialist readership. Ruth R. Levine's *Pharmacology: Drug Actions and*

Reactions, 6th ed. (New York & London: The Parthenon Publishing Group, 2000) provides a less detailed exposition in Chap. 3, pp. 27–49. T.Z. Csáky's *Introduction to General Pharmacology* (New York: Appleton-Century Crofts, 1979), Part I, Chaps. 3 and 5 give a readable student account of the topic.

2. A brief biography of A.J. Clark can be found in B. Holmstedt and G. Liljestrand (eds.), *Readings in Pharmacology* (1963), p. 270 (see also Note 2 under Chap. 16).

3. *Microiontophoresis* is a highly sensitive modification of the technique of iontophoresis in which the ions of a drug, transmitter, etc., are introduced into the tissues by means of an electric current. *Patch clamping* is a technique to study the electrical properties of the ion channels in receptors, and how they are regulated by neurotransmitters. See *Goodman and Gilman* (2001), Chap. 12, p. 301.

4. See Solomon H. Snyder, *Brainstorming: The Science and Politics of Opiate Research* (Cambridge MA and London: Harvard University Press, 1989), pp. 113–16.

Chapter 14

1. Much of the material in this chapter is derived from the following books: Mary Kilbourne Matossian, *Poisons of the Past: Molds, Epidemics and History*, (New Haven: Yale University Press, 1989); Richard P. Wedeen, *Poison in the Pot: The Legacy of Lead* (Carbondale, IL: Southern Illinois University Press, 1984); and Jerome O. Nriagu, *Lead and Lead Poisoning in Antiquity* (New York: John Wiley & Sons, Inc., 1983).

2. Thomas Hobbes (1588–1679), *Leviathan*, Part 1, Chap. XIII.

3. Aluminium hydroxide (as Aludrox) is still widely used as an antacid and for the relief of gastric irritation. Industrial waste containing large amounts of aluminium was dumped into a reservoir in Cornwall, UK some years ago, but long-term toxic effects were not observed.

4. Oil firms were aware of the toxic health effects of leaded petrol as long ago as the 1920s, but denied them to preserve their lucrative monopoly. See *Guardian Weekly*, Vol. 163, No. 4 (20–26 July 2000).

5. See "Anthropogenic Lead in Greenland", *Nature*, Vol. 353 (12 September 1991), p. 189.

Chapter 15

1. Brief descriptions of Minamata Disease and Itai-itai Disease can be found in *Goodman and Gilman* (2001), pp. 1865, 1867 and 1958; and in David Day, *The Environmental Wars: Reports from the Front Line* (New York: St. Martin's

Press, 1989), pp. 211–12. *Itai-itai* is said to be translatable as 'ouch-ouch', no doubt referring to the severe pain caused by the typical osteomalacia!

2. David Weir and Mark Schapiro, *The Circle of Poison: Pesticides and People in a Hungry World*, (San Francisco: Institute for Food and Development Policy, 1981).

3. Professor S. Feldman, Personal Communication.

4. Don Kurzman, *A Killing Wind: Inside Union Carbide and the Bhopal Catastrophe* (New York: McGraw-Hill, 1987).

5. See Thomas Whiteside, *The Pendulum and the Toxic Cloud: The Course of Dioxin Contamination* (New Haven: Yale University Press, 1979). A brief reference to the Seveso Disaster is found in David Day, *The Environmental Wars* (1989), pp. 193–94.

6. More recent follow-up findings were quoted in *Scientific American* (January 1994). People living in the second most polluted area, but not evacuated at the time of the disaster, were three times more likely to develop liver cancer. Females were 5.3 times more likely to get a form of myeloma, and 5.7 times more likely to develop blood cancers. The article suggests that dioxin functions as a hormone and affects the immune system and the reproductive tract, and acts as a potent growth factor.

7. See Jerome O. Nriagu (ed.), *Arsenic in the Environment* (New York: John Wiley & Sons, Inc., 1994).

Part II

Chapter 16

1. Professor S. Feldman, Personal Communication.

2. Much of the material in Chaps. 16–19 on the history of early pharmacology, especially the development of theories of chemical transmission in the ANS, is taken from B. Holmstedt and G. Liljestrand (eds.), *Readings in Pharmacology* (1963). This interesting and unusual book includes extracts from seminal publications, together with brief biographical accounts and pictures of leading investigators in the field.

Chapter 18

1. For more on betel nut and its preparations, see *Goodman and Gilman* (2001), p. 159; and *Ellenhorn's Medical Toxicology: Diagnosis and Treatment of Human Poisoning*, 2nd ed. (Baltimore: Williams and Wilkins, 1997), p. 1823.

2. *The Lancet*, Vol. 341 (27 March 1993), p. 818 reported this warning by the Indian government about the carcinogenic effects of "panmasala", a powdered and concentrated preparation containing betel nut.

Chapter 19

1. See *Goodman and Gilman* (2001), pp. 227–35.
2. See B. Holmstedt and G. Liljestrand (eds.), *Readings in Pharmacology* (1963), Chap. XI, pp. 342–48.

Chapter 20

1. B. Holmstedt and G. Liljestrand (eds.), *Readings in Pharmacology* (1963), Chap. VI, p. 202. This whole chapter provides an interesting historical survey of the beginnings of neuropharmacology.
2. Solomon H. Snyder, *Brainstorming: The Science and Politics of Opiate Research* (1989), p. 111. Snyder's actual words were: "Located far in the north of Scotland, Aberdeen was virtually inaccessible in 1933, physically as well as intellectually."
3. Snyder's pioneering work on opiate and dopamine receptors in the brain, and elsewhere in the body, is summarized in his book *Brainstorming: The Science and Politics of Opiate Research* (1989).

Chapter 21

1. For example, see Niall Quin, "Fortnightly Review: Drug Treatment of Parkinson's Disease" *BMJ*, Vol. 310 (4 March 1995), pp. 575–79.
2. For the views of S.H. Snyder, see his book *Brainstorming: The Science and Politics of Opiate Research* (1989), Chap. 9, especially pp. 177–79.

Chapter 22

1. Aldous Huxley, *The Doors of Perception* (London: Chatto and Windus, 1954).
2. Louis Lewin, *Phantastica: Narcotic and Stimulating Drugs, Their Use and Abuse*, with a foreword by B. Holmstedt (New York: E.P. Dutton & Co., Inc., 1964).
3. A very recent book (2000) on this topic is Mike Jay, *Emperors of Dreams: Drugs in the Nineteenth Century* (Dedalus Ltd., Langford Lodge, St. Judith's Lane, Sawtry, Cambs. PE17 6XB). He "tells the stories of how all these substances [cannabis, cocaine, opium, ether, mescaline] were first discovered … " He shows that "the age of Empire and Victorian values was awash with legal narcotics, stimulants and psychedelics … "
4. Heffter's account of mescaline self-administration is taken from B. Holmstedt and G. Liljestrand (eds.), *Readings in Pharmacology* (1963), Chap. VI, pp. 207–209.
5. See B. Holmstedt and G. Liljestrand (eds.), *Readings in Pharmacology* (1963) Chap. VI, pp. 210–13.

6. From *The Alice B. Toklas Cook Book* (1954), quoted by D.R. Laurence and P. N. Bennett in *Clinical Pharmacology* (1980), p. 499.
7. From John R. Milton (ed.), *Conversations with Frank Waters* (Chicago: The Swallow Press Inc., 1971), Chap. 7, pp. 81–85.

Chapter 23

1. See S.H. Snyder, *Brainstorming: The Science and Politics of Opiate Research* (1989), Chap. 9, pp. 166–74.
2. Cocaine is another drug which blocks the re-uptake transport system for noradrenaline at the adrenergic nerve terminal. See *Goodman and Gilman* (2001), p. 144.

Chapter 24

1. Thomas S. Szasz, *The Manufacture of Madness*, (New York: Delta Book, 1970).
2. Richard Hughes and Robert Brewin, *The Tranquilizing of America: Pill Popping and the American Way of Life* (New York & London: Harcourt Brace Jovanovitch, 1979), Chaps. 5 and 6, pp. 142–89.

Chapter 25

1. Thomas S. Szasz, *The Myth of Mental Illness: Foundations of a Theory of Personal Conduct*, revised ed. (Harper and Row, New York, Evanstown, San Francisco, London, 1974).
2. Thomas Szasz, "Diagnoses are not Diseases", *The Lancet*, Vol. 338 (21/28 December 1991), pp. 1574–76.
3. *Diagnostic and Statistical Manual of Mental Disorders*, 4th ed. (Washington, DC: American Psychiatric Association, 2000).
4. Garth Wood, *The Myth of Neurosis: A Case for Moral Therapy* (London: Macmillan, 1984). See also Richard Hughes and Robert Brewin's depressing account of tranquillizer-addiction in the USA in *The Tranquilizing of America* (1979), Chaps. 1 and 2. See also "The Risks of Tranquility", *Health Letter*, Vol. 16, No. 8 (August 2000) (Public Citizen Health Research Group), pp. 9–10.

Chapter 26

1. *BMJ*, Vol. 297 (16 November 1988), p. 1415.
2. Wallace B. Mendelson, *Human Sleep: Research and Clinical Care* (New York and London: Plenum Medical Book Co., 1987), Chaps. 1, 2 and 12, from which much of the material in this chapter is taken

3. Electrically induced sleep can be produced in man, and this technique was tried out for surgical procedures by French surgeons between 1970 and 1980. It was abandoned because muscle relaxation did not occur. (Professor S. Feldman, Personal Communication).
4. See *Goodman and Gilman* (2001), p. 270, for more about melatonin.
5. See under the title *Dangerous Diets* in the Notes and News Section of *The Lancet* (16 December, 1989), p. 1466.

Chapter 27

1. For a full discussion of tolerance, dependence and withdrawal syndromes, mentioned in this and later chapters, see "Drug Addiction and Drug Abuse", *Goodman and Gilman* (2001), Chap. 24.
2. See Note 4, Chap. 25.
3. *BMJ*, Vol. 305 (19 September 1992), p. 672.

Chapter 28

1. A useful and informative book is Charles B. Spacy, Andrew S. Kaplan and Gray Williams, *The Fight Against Pain* (Yonkers, New York: Computer Reports Books, 1992).
2. D.R. Laurence and P.N. Bennett, *Clinical Pharmacology* (1980), p. 422. The figures quoted are taken from an Editorial in *The Lancet* (1972), p. 477.
3. See J.R. Vane and R. M. Botting, "Inflammation and the Mechanism of Action of Anti-inflammatory Drugs", *FASEB J.*, Vol 1 (1987), pp. 89–96; and J.R. Vane and R.M. Botting, "New Insights into the Mode of Action of Anti-inflammatory Drugs", *Inflamm. Res.*, Vol 44 (1995), pp. 1–10.
4. Cocaine was isolated in 1858 from *Erythroxylon coca* by A. Niemann in the laboratory of F. Wöhler, who reported the discovery in 1860. Carl Koller introduced its use as an anaesthetic in 1884.
5. The biblical comment that "man is born in pain" was falsely interpreted to mean that pain should never be alleviated! The famous English physician Thomas Sydenham wrote in 1680: "Among the remedies which it has pleased Almighty God to give to man to relieve his sufferings, none is so universal and so efficacious as opium."
6. See Solomon H. Snyder, *Brainstorming: The Science and Politics of Opiate Research* (1989), pp. 86–89.
7. Further details of the properties and uses of the more recent analgesic and anaesthetic drugs can be found in *Goodman and Gilman* (2001): e.g. propofol, pp. 344–45; buprenorphine, pp. 601–602; fentanyl and alfentanil, pp. 595–96; and clonidine and dexmedetomidine, p. 358.
8. The story of FK-33824 is told by S.H. Snyder in his *Brainstorming: The Science and Politics of Opiate Research* (1989), pp. 141–43.

Chapter 29

1. The mildly stimulant drug methylphenidate (Ritalin) is chemically related to amphetamine, but has the paradoxical property of sedating hyperactive children. It has acquired much notoriety for being widely prescribed in the USA to overactive children who cannot concentrate in the classroom and generally disturb their fellow pupils. The condition is known as Attention-Deficit Hyperactivity Disorder (ADHD). Is this a genuine psychological disorder, or the medicalization of mere excessive youthful exuberance? See *Goodman and Gilman* (2001), p. 241 for more about ADHD and p. 237 for more about Ritalin.

Chapter 30

1. For a full account of the pharmacology of disulfiram and its use in treating alcoholism, see *Goodman and Gilman* (2001), pp. 441–42.
2. V.P. Dole and M. Nyswander, "A Medical Treatment for Heroin Addiction: A Clinical Trial with Methadone Hydrochloride", *JAMA*, Vol. 193 (1965), p. 80.
3. Joyce H. Lowinson and Pedro Ruiz (eds.), *Substance Abuse: Clinical Problems and Perspectives* (Baltimore and London: Williams and Wilkins, 1981). See "Methadone Maintenance in Perspective", Chap. 26, p. 344, which concludes: "Although methadone maintenance is not a panacea for narcotic addiction — and never promised to be — its contribution to successful treatment is undeniable. It remains a very useful tool in our treatment armamentarium."

Chapter 31

1. This must have been true of opium smoking, too, in past times; and even recently in some parts of the world. Professor S. Feldman saw many opium addicts in Tehran over 70 years of age who suffered from chronic bronchitis, and were liable to die of respiratory depression if they contracted lung infections (Professor S. Feldman, Personal Communication).
2. For further information, see J.D.P. Graham (ed.), *Cannabis and Health* (London, New York & San Francisco: Academic Press, 1976).
3. "Ritual" is the key word here. *Homo sapiens*' highly developed cerebral cortex enables him to manipulate symbols and concepts, and thereby escape the constraints of instinctual behaviour. The evolutionary pay-off is a mental freedom that animals do not share; but at the same time it leads to the burden and anxiety of choice, and the dangers of license and loss of control. Ritual, along with custom and taboo, have come to play important societal roles in checking these outcomes. Mind-altering drugs, with which man has been

familiar since prehistoric times, can pose one such threat, and over time ritualistic methods of controlling their use have evolved. To legalize a drug unfamiliar to Western use (e.g. cannabis), though it may not be any more deleterious than the already acceptable drugs, could court disaster. A lesson can be learnt from the socially destructive results of the introduction by Europeans of alcoholic liquors to aboriginal tribes in many parts of the world. The problem of drug abuse is not just a pharmacological one; it is a psychological and a spiritual problem too.

4. Virginia Berridge and Griffith Edwards, *Opium and the People: Opiate Use in Nineteenth-Century England* (New Haven & London: Yale University Press, 1987).

5. From Charles Kingsley, *Alton Locke* (London 1850), quoted by Virginia Berridge and Griffith Edwards, *Opium and the People: Opiate Use in Nineteenth-Century England* (1987), p. 42.

6. See the leading article "Artificial Paradises Encapsulated" in *The Lancet*, Vol. 343, No. 8902 (9 April 1994), p. 865.

Index